D0141927

THE BATTLE AGAINST BACTERIA

A HISTORY OF THE DEVELOPMENT OF ANTIBACTERIAL DRUGS, FOR THE GENERAL READER

BY

P. E. BALDRY

M.B., B.S., M.R.C.P.

*Consultant Physician, Ashford General Hospital, Middlesex,
St Mary's Cottage Hospital, Hampton, and The Memorial
Hospital, Teddington, Middlesex*

CAMBRIDGE
AT THE UNIVERSITY PRESS
1965

PUBLISHED BY
THE SYNDICS OF THE CAMBRIDGE UNIVERSITY PRESS

Bentley House, 200 Euston Road, London, N.W. 1
American Branch: 32 East 57th Street, New York, N.Y. 10022
West African Office: P.O. Box 33, Ibadan, Nigeria

©

CAMBRIDGE UNIVERSITY PRESS
1965

Printed in Great Britain at the University Printing House, Cambridge
(Brooke Crutchley, University Printer)

LIBRARY OF CONGRESS CATALOGUE
CARD NUMBER: 65-15311

QR
46
.B28

To
NORMAN MATHESON,
F.R.C.S., F.R.A.C.S., M.R.C.P.
without whose encouragement this book would not
have been written

CONTENTS

Plates 1–8 appear between pages 38 and 39

...in the field of experiment, chance favours only the prepared mind.

LOUIS PASTEUR

PREFACE

Until the end of the last century there was a great risk of dying from some microbial disease before reaching the age of forty. A large number of people succumbed in infancy or childhood and others in early adult life. Now, thanks to scientific advances made in the last fifty years, death for most people in Western countries has been deferred and they have a very good chance of enjoying their full span of years. The proportion of old people in our midst today is higher than ever before and this is largely due to the recent success in the fight against microbes. As a practising physician it has been my privilege to take part in this battle and to use some of the powerful weapons at our disposal. They have brought about such a great change in the pattern of disease that I was prompted to inquire how they were discovered, and a story so dramatic and full of such interest was revealed to me, that it is the purpose of this book to share it with others.

My sincere thanks are due to Miss K. M. Young for her invaluable help in the preparation of the manuscript and to the editorial staff of the Cambridge University Press for kindly reading the text and making many helpful suggestions. I also gratefully acknowledge the advice of Dr F. N. L. Poynter, Director and formerly Chief Librarian of the Wellcome Historical Medical Library, and Mr Alistair Warren of Messrs Alex. Cowan and Sons, Ltd.

P. E. B.

1

THE UNKNOWN ENEMY

Mankind has always been affected by disease which at times, in the form of pestilence or plague, has spread throughout entire communities. These epidemics were originally believed to be visitations by the gods intended to punish evil doers, although the mechanism by which the wrath of the gods produced this terrible effect remained unexplained. Hippocrates, the famous Greek physician, born in 460 B.C., firmly rejected this notion. A very observant man with a clear logical mind who, during the course of a long distinguished career, formulated precepts, aphorisms and laws which have had an important influence on medical thought ever since. He believed that ill health arose from external earthly causes such as cold, sun or changing winds. He noted the effect of food, occupation and climate on the causation of disease, and one of his best known books, *Airs, Waters and Places*, deals with the influence of climate, prevailing winds, water supplies, the nature of the soil and the habits of the people, on the illnesses from which they suffered. Although time has shown that these factors are of undoubted importance, it was soon obvious that they did not afford a complete explanation of the origin and spread of disease. It had long been observed that disease could be transmitted from one person to another when in close proximity and could also be spread by clothing or objects in common use. This led physicians to postulate that disease was caused by animated particles invisible to the naked eye. This theory was clearly expressed by Varro (117–26 B.C.) when he stated that disease was caused by tiny animals which could not be seen by the naked eye but which were carried with the air through the mouth and nose into the body. Similarly the early Teutons are said to have pictured minute worm-like creatures coming out of the nostrils, eyes and ears of sick individuals and passing into the bodies of others. Thus at a very early stage man developed a concept that contagious disease was caused by invisible living things, but it was not until the invention of the microscope that the idea could be shown to be a reality. In the meantime, however, general measures were taken to prevent the spread of contagious disease.

The ancient Hebrews recognized that leprosy was readily transmitted from one person to another and devised regulations to prevent its spread, which may be found in the thirteenth and fourteenth chapters of the book of Leviticus. Explicit instructions to be observed by the priest included the isolation of the patient, the washing and burning of infected clothing, and the disinfection of houses—if necessary their complete destruction. Strict enforcement of similar rules continued throughout many parts of the world up to the Middle Ages, so that lepers were driven out of the community away from families and friends, and forced to live in abandoned places and to subsist largely on charity. The unfortunate sufferer was made to announce his approach by shaking a bell or rattle or by blowing a horn and crying 'Unclean'. Governments also instituted compulsory medical inspection of the population and anyone deemed to be suffering from the disease was deprived of his property and pronounced legally dead. As we look back upon these practices today they appear to be unnecessarily harsh and cruel; nevertheless, they were the first steps in public health control and did demonstrate that, in order to prevent the spread of disease in a community, it is necessary for its members to conform to certain regulations.

Plague was another disease for which rules were made to prevent its spread, long before the causative organism was recognized. It is a horrible condition which may cause large swellings in the groin and armpits, or seriously affect the lungs. The disease spread from the East and from A.D. 900 to 1500 it attacked Europe sixty-five times. The serious epidemic in the fourteenth century known as the Black Death began as usual in the Far East, where millions died in India and China, and spread to Europe in 1347, first to Italy, then to France and finally to England. In an attempt to check it in Venice a detention hospital was opened in 1403 on an island adjoining the city, for the isolation of all travellers from the Levant for a period of 30 to 40 days. The period of 40 days was apparently chosen because at that stage of world history religious ideas were dominant and that particular length of time had great biblical significance. It was from this regulation that our term 'quarantine' arose.

In 1467 a similar hospital was opened in Genoa, and in 1476 the authorities in Marseilles converted their old leper hospital into a plague hospital. By this time leprosy was so well under control that hospitals set aside for its management could be converted for use against this further health hazard. This practice of isolation and detention of travellers in order to see whether or not they were incubating the plague soon became world wide and helped to establish the general principle that transmittable diseases may be controlled by removing the sufferer from the community.

Syphilis is a further example of a disease which was known to be contagious long before the causative organism was identified. At the beginning of the sixteenth century sufficient was known about it to make diagnosis easy and, since it was realized that it was transmitted by sexual intercourse, various preventive measures could be taken to stop its spread. The disease first hit Europe with a forceful and devastating impact towards the end of the fifteenth century, when it was far more acute than at the present time. It was characterized by widespread skin eruptions and ulcers, with much destruction of tissue, which often led to death. The speed with which it reached epidemic proportions soon attracted the attention of physicians and led them to make it the subject of special study. There has been much controversy regarding the part of the world in which syphilis originated, one theory being that the sailors of Columbus, having been infected by the natives in Haiti, brought it back to the Spanish occupants of Naples. There is evidence however to show that it was in Europe before the discovery of America. A further theory is that it was brought to Europe by sailors landing on the south coast of Spain after returning from voyages to West Africa; the exact truth will probably never be known. There seems little doubt that the disease ravaged the army of Charles VIII of France during the siege of Naples in 1495 and was disseminated widely by his band of mercenaries on their return to France, so the French called it the Neapolitan disease while the Spaniards always referred to it as the French disease. It was the Italian physician Fracastorius (1483–1553) who put an end to the argument by giving it the name of syphilis. He was especially interested in diseases which spread from one person to another and had made a study of leprosy and plague, both of which by his time, as has been shown, were controlled by isolation of the victim and destruction of contaminated objects. When a new type of disease which seemed to be passed from one person to another during sexual intercourse appeared in the neighbourhood, he quickly became interested. After a period of study he became inspired to write a poem about it in Latin hexameter! Turning to Ovid to find a name for a central character his choice fell upon Syphilus, the second son of Niobe. In his poem, Syphilus, a shepherd boy, because of an act of impiety, brought down upon him the anger of the sun god and was given as a punishment a loathsome and contagious disease. The poem became famous and it was from the name of this mythical character that the disease received its title. He published the results of his studies on these three contagious diseases, leprosy, plague and syphilis, in a famous book *De Contagione*, in 1546. He postulated that certain diseases were transmitted by imperceptible particles which he called *seminaria contagionum* or the 'seeds of disease', and considered that this could happen either by direct contact with the sick person, or by contact with his clothing or utensils, or in some cases by the 'seeds' being carried through the air. His concept was extraordinarily clear, although formulated centuries before it could be proved that certain diseases are spread by bacteria. His book was a most valuable contribution to knowledge about the control of infectious diseases and, because of it, he has the right to be regarded as the father of modern epidemiology.

In addition to passing laws about individual diseases, the human race was quick to appreciate the value of general rules of hygiene, as is again shown in the Old Testament. A good example appears in Deuteronomy, chapter xxiii, verse 13, where Moses gives instructions that every soldier shall carry a spade in order to bury his excreta so as not to defile the camp—'and thou shalt have a paddle upon thy weapon; and it shall be, when thou wilt ease thyself abroad, thou shalt dig therewith, and shalt turn back and cover that which cometh from thee'. The disposal of sewage in big towns is obviously a far more difficult problem, but unfortunately those in authority have not always been sufficiently strict in the matter. This applied in Great Britain up to the nineteenth century and is still true in certain parts of the world. Because of this lack of insistence on proper sanitation, there were serious widespread epidemics of cholera, typhoid and dysentery in Europe up to the middle of the last century. The description of conditions in big cities at that time showed that the filth was appalling. In the tenements of Glasgow dung was left lying in the courtyards adjacent to the houses as there were no drains or privies; in another Scottish town it was reported that there were no lavatories in houses and only two or three public privies, situated in the better parts of the town. These two examples were typical of the situation in all big cities. This lack of lavatories either public or private led to the habit of house dwellers filling chamber pots with excreta and after some days, when completely full, and with a shout of 'Gardez l'eau', emptying the contents out of the window into the street below; a habit not without risk to passers by, and of course a practice which led to persistent pollution and stench in all the streets. The lawyer Edwin Chadwick (1800–90) attempted to reform these conditions, producing in 1842 the well known report on the sanitary conditions of the labouring population in Great Britain in which he pointed out that much disease could be prevented by proper drainage, the removal of refuse from houses and streets, and the improvement of water supplies.

Doubt as to whether excreta alone could cause disease however was already present in the minds of thinking people before germs were identified under the microscope. William Budd, the great epidemiologist of the nineteenth century, took the opportunity of the famous Great Stench of London, which occurred during the summer months of 1858, to point out that organic putrefaction by itself was not enough to cause disease. At that time, the sewage of nearly three million people was allowed to collect in one vast cess-pit in the middle of the city, and during the summer the hot sun shining on this quagmire produced a stench so foul as had never been experienced before. The work of Parliament was almost brought to a standstill because of the noxious air which penetrated the building, and steps were taken to overcome this by the suspension before every window of blankets saturated in chloride of lime, and by the lavish use of this and other disinfectants in every room. The Law Courts had to close down and travellers who could do so avoided London by making a wide detour of the city. The newspapers were full of letters from anxious members of the public about the stench, some prophesying calamity, others suggesting remedies; it became the most frequent topic of conversation, everyone convinced that it would be followed by a widespread and devastating epidemic of disease. People were amazed to find that as the season passed there was in fact a remarkable diminution in the proportion of fevers, diarrhoea and other forms of disease which had commonly been attributed to decaying dung. It was obvious therefore that this had to contain some additional poison to make it harmful, a fact which had already been shown to be true by some observations made by John Snow in 1854, during the last great cholera epidemic in Great Britain. He considered that cholera, a disease in which there is profuse and watery diarrhoea, was due to a poison taken into the mouth with excreta from some other sufferer. He believed that this could happen if contaminated water was used for drinking, and proved this theory by studying a large number of outbreaks and by paying special attention in every instance to the water supply. At first his teaching was ignored, until he was able to present striking supporting evidence at the time of a dramatic outbreak of the disease in Broad Street, London. In this epidemic 500 people living within two hundred yards of where the first case was diagnosed, died of the disease within the incredibly short period of ten days. The rest of the inhabitants of the street not unnaturally took fright and hurriedly left. Snow was able to show that all the victims used a pump connected to one particular well and that a person suffering from cholera had been in the habit of using a certain cesspool which he found drained into this well. As soon as he put the pump out of action by removing the handle no further case occurred. Although he was not able to demonstrate the micro-organism responsible for cholera, he established by inference that the disease is spread by water which has been contaminated by excreta containing some noxious agent.

There was therefore good evidence by the middle of the last century that some diseases are spread by air and some by water, while others like syphilis and leprosy are spread by the direct contact of one person with another. In addition it was becoming recognized that it was possible for a healthy person to be the carrier of germs and to spread them to other people causing them to become ill. This was perhaps best demonstrated in the maternity hospitals where it was found that a very high percentage of women admitted to hospital for the birth of their babies developed an overwhelming and usually fatal form of blood poisoning some days afterwards. This feverish illness, because it occurred in the puerperium, was called puerperal fever and it is reported that out of 9886 pregnant women who were confined in the maternity hospital in Paris between 1861 and 1864, 1226 died of this disease. The situation was similarly bad in all the lying-in hospitals in Europe and other parts of the world. Oliver Wendell Holmes of Boston taught, in 1843, that puerperal fever was caused by germs on the hands of physicians and midwives carried into the bodies of these unfortunate women during internal examinations. There was much opposition to this theory, for the medical profession resented the implication that physicians were not clean, and his warning was not heeded in America for a long time. Semmelweis taught the same principle in the maternity hospital in Vienna, but was similarly ignored. He realized that the medical students often came straight to the maternity wards after dealing with highly infectious patients in other wards, as well as after dissecting dead bodies in the post-mortem room. He therefore made it a strict rule that all students should wash their hands in a solution of chloride of lime before carrying out internal examinations on women, and by this means the mortality rate on his wards fell from 18 per cent to only 1 per cent. In spite of this remarkable success he was scorned, persecuted and forced to resign his position as professor, and moved to Budapest where in 1861 he published his book *The Cause and Prevention of Puerperal Fever*, but he never convinced his critics. He became insane and died from a septic wound of the hand, a tragic ending for a man whose teaching has since been proved correct.

It may be seen therefore that observant men were able to gain much knowledge about the spread and control of certain diseases long before the causative germs were identified under the microscope.

2

THE ENEMY IDENTIFIED

It is thought that a knowledge of lenses developed about the time of Euclid in the third century B.C. and that Ptolemy of Alexandria (about A.D. 150) was probably the first to study the laws of refraction of light. In England, the Franciscan friar Roger Bacon (1214–94) did much work with lenses and clearly set out the laws of refraction and reflection; he also suggested the use of lenses to improve vision. Leonardo da Vinci, in the fifteenth century, was well acquainted with the use of lenses, and Zacharias Jansen, a Dutch spectacle maker, about 1609, accidentally discovered the principle of the telescope and microscope by placing two lenses together in a tube.

The first to apply this invention to medicine was Professor Kircher (1602–80), a Jesuit priest and doctor of Würzburg. He examined the blood of patients suffering from plague, and reported that through the microscope he saw countless masses of small worms invisible to the naked eye. It has since been generally agreed that he was really only looking at red blood cells as the magnification available in his day would not have been sufficient to show the tiny germs which cause plague. Nevertheless he must be given credit for having made the correct deduction that a contagious disease was caused by microscopic organisms.

The greatest of all early microscopists was Antony Van Leeuwenhoek (1632–1723), a Dutch draper, whose interest in microscopes started as a hobby early in his life. He made a large number of them and at his death bequeathed twenty-six lenses set in silver to the Royal Society of London. He made several observations by looking down the microscope and was the first to show that the red cells in the blood of men are round, whereas in fish and amphibians they are oval. He also described many of the microscopic organisms seen in stagnant pond life but his most important achievement, from the medical point of view, was that he was the first to see the little animalcules, as he called them, which cause disease. His demonstrations of bacteria were made public by letters to the Royal Society between 1675 and 1685. He made detailed observations of the bacteria to be found in the mouth by examining the deposit which collected round his teeth and he said that he saw 'little animals more numerous than all the people in the Netherlands and moving about in the most delightful manner'. Although many people at that time considered that animalcules such as Leeuwenhoek described might well be the cause of contagious disease, it was not for another two hundred years that this idea was finally accepted and firmly established as a scientific fact.

Marcus Plenciz, a Viennese physician, in his *Opera Medico-Physica* published in 1762, clearly expressed the opinion that infectious diseases were spread through the air by contagious animalcules, though he was unable to put forward any proof of this. Probably the first man to present real evidence that living organisms were the cause of disease was Bassi, who in 1836, after working for years on a certain disease which affects silkworms, was able to demonstrate that it was caused by a fungus which could be transmitted from one worm to another. No definite evidence about the part played by bacteria in the production of disease could however be obtained until a large number of different micro-organisms had been identified. An important contribution to this was made by Ehrenberg (1795–1876), who was able to distinguish between various types of micro-organisms and to place them in a simple classification. His task was made easier by using a technique, introduced by Wilhelm von Gleichen, of staining the organisms with powdered carmine or indigo. Scientists sought hard to find microbes in diseased tissue in order to be able to prove the microbial cause of infective disease, but many were carried away by their enthusiasm and made rash statements based on slipshod and uncritical work. This led the anatomist Jacob Henle to write an essay in 1840 in which he protested vigorously against certain ill-founded conclusions. He stated that before any microscopic organism could be regarded as a cause of disease in man, it must be found constantly in the diseased tissue, it must be isolated from it, and it must be possible to reproduce the disease with it. These clear principles were to influence greatly two men, Louis Pasteur and Robert Koch, who twenty years later were able to place the germ theory of disease on a sound scientific basis.

Louis Pasteur came from a humble home. His father, who had been a sergeant in Napoleon's army, was working as a tanner in the little town of Dole in Southern France when Louis was born in 1822. He was a conscientious lad, but there was nothing to make him stand out from others except, in his teens, a proficiency in portrait painting and, as a student, a determination that one day he would become a professor himself. After he qualified he asked the famous chemist Jean Dumas to employ him as a teaching assistant because, as he said, he had the ambition to become a distinguished professor; to a friend he wrote 'those of us who are to become professors must make the art of teaching our chief concern'—an extremely praiseworthy attitude, all too often lacking in men of great academic attainment. He proved himself to be an excellent teacher, but was not content merely to pass on knowledge obtained by others; he also had an innate drive to make original discoveries.

He was fortunate as a student in having the stimulating influence of two great chemists, Dumas and Antoine Balard. Dumas, a dynamic teacher, was to remain an inspiration to Pasteur all his life. Balard was a colourful, if somewhat eccentric, chemist who, even after he achieved success, lived in a shabby room furnished with two shaky armchairs which he painted a peculiar red colour under the illusion that it made them look as if they were made of mahogany! He was nevertheless a man of great ability, who took a deep personal interest in his student, and encouraged him to spend his spare time doing chemical experiments in his laboratory. Pasteur took good advantage of this and it was there that before long he made important fundamental contributions to the science of crystallography.

After Pasteur passed his examinations his tutors were very anxious for him to stay in Paris, but a decision was made by the Minister of Education to send him elsewhere to take up a teaching post. First, he was given a junior post at Dijon in 1847, but after a few months he was sent as acting professor of chemistry at the University of Strasbourg. This was a happy choice because it brought him into contact with Pierre Bertin-Mourot, professor of physics at the University in whose house he stayed. This physicist was not only an able scientist and teacher, but also had a great capacity to enjoy life, and introduced the serious-minded, intense, humourless young scholar to some of the simple pleasures of living, inculcating in him an appreciation of good wine and beer, which surprisingly enough, as will be seen, was to be a great asset to him before long in his professional life. It was also at Strasbourg that he met Marie Laurent, the daughter of the university rector, who was to share a long and happy life with him after their marriage in 1849. Pasteur's approach to the gentleman whose daughter he wished to marry was simple and direct; he wrote to him explaining that he had no money, but was imbued with good health, courage and a position in the university. He added that he had held a doctor's degree for eighteen months and had presented a few pieces of original work to the Academy of Science which had been well received. He then took the somewhat unusual step, for a suitor seeking to commend himself to a prospective father-in-law, of enclosing a report of an investigation which he had recently presented to a learned society!

The course of his life was again changed by a decree of the Minister of Education, when in 1854 he was appointed professor of chemistry at Lille, with the recommendation that he centred his teaching and research round the problems of the local industries. One of the main industries in this city was the fermentation of beet sugar to produce alcohol, and surprisingly, it was a study of this that led Pasteur to an understanding of the part played by microbes in the production of disease. Shortly after arriving at Lille he was asked to investigate certain difficulties experienced in this particular industry which led Marie Pasteur to complain, in a letter to her father, that 'Louis spends all his days in the distillery and is up to his neck in beet juice!'

The term fermentation was used in those days to describe the process by which spiritous or acid substances were obtained from organic liquids, but it was not known how this took place. Thus the production of alcohol from beet juice was called alcoholic fermentation; the conversion of wine into vinegar was called acetic acid fermentation; and the souring of milk, during which lactic acid is produced, was called lactic acid fermentation. It was thought that the fermentation of liquids was possibly brought about by changes similar to those which occurred in meat or eggs during decomposition and putrefaction. The great chemists of that time, such as Lavoisier,

Gay-Lussac, Thénard and Dumas, taught that all changes in organic substances could be readily explained in terms of chemical reactions and expressed by means of chemical formulae. Lavoisier was therefore content to explain the production of alcohol from carbohydrate by stating that the latter split into two parts and that, by transfer of oxygen from one part to another, alcohol was formed. This failed to explain what made the carbohydrate undergo this change, and also ignored the fact that yeast always had to be present for it to take place. This substance had been known since primitive man used it not only to change starch into bread, but also to produce alcoholic liquids from sugar solutions.

In the 1830's it was shown that yeast was not simply an organic substance, but was made up of living cells which, under the microscope, could be observed to multiply by budding. Many people considered that alcoholic fermentation must depend on the presence and action of these living cells, but the leading chemists, including Liebig, did everything possible to discredit this theory. Liebig was willing to concede that yeast may be a small plant, but considered that, if it made any contribution to alcoholic fermentation, it was not during life, but only after death, when its protein imparted a vibration to the sugar molecule causing it to break down, with the production of alcohol. As Pasteur had been trained as a chemist it would have been easy for him to conform to these current orthodox opinions, but to his eternal credit he would not be dominated by his teachers and, seeing the weakness in their theories, was determined to discover the truth. He confirmed, by well designed experiments, that the production of alcohol from sugar was brought about by the action of yeast cells and that the amount of alcohol produced was directly proportional to the number of cells present. He had previously shown that a grey material, made out of living cells which were smaller but otherwise similar to yeast cells, was sometimes found in milk, and that this material acted as a ferment turning the milk sour with the production of lactic acid.

He next studied the manufacture of vinegar. It was well known that vinegar was produced by the oxidation of alcohol, a process which at that time was considered to be purely chemical. In France, alcohol was allowed to undergo this oxidation in casks standing on end, while the German process consisted of pouring a mixture of alcohol, acetic acid and beer over a hollow column, several metres high, of loosely piled beech shavings. These two well-known processes had been devised many years previously in an empirical manner without anyone knowing why they worked, although Liebig considered he could explain the mechanism in both cases on the basis of organic chemical reactions. He ignored however the fact that the French workers in Orleans had observed that a fragile skin or pellicle always formed on the surface of the liquid in the casks, and that for the change from wine to vinegar to take place this pellicle had to remain intact. It was for this reason that the skin was known as 'the mother of vinegar'. When in 1837 Kutzing demonstrated that it was made up of living cells, some people concluded that these cells must be responsible for the essential chemical change. The chemists were not willing to consider this idea, but Pasteur felt it was worth further investigation, and was able to prove in the laboratory that the microscopic cells present in the thin skin covering the wine were responsible for its conversion into vinegar. He was also able to detect a barely visible film of organisms on the surface of the wood shavings used in the German process, and showed that if these shavings were heated, the organisms were destroyed and the shavings were then useless for their purpose. He was thus able to supply a clear explanation for this well established technique and to recommend certain alterations which enabled the manufacture of vinegar to become more efficient.

Pasteur's work on the production of lactic acid, alcohol and vinegar was of great fundamental importance for, from this, scientists had to accept that changes in organic material could be brought about by microscopic organisms.

His next step was to demonstrate the adverse effect which certain microbes could have on the fermentation of wine and beer. He published his findings in a book about wine in 1866. His interest in the subject started while he was on holiday at Arbois in 1858, for it was there that he examined samples of Jura wines under the microscope and saw living cells in them similar to the lactic acid organisms he had observed in sour milk. This observation, together with his experiments in the distilleries, led him to conclude that fermentation of wine could be disturbed by other organisms competing with yeast.

A friend at Arbois then asked him to examine microscopically a selection of good and sour wines and he was able to demonstrate various micro-organisms amongst the yeast cells in the spoiled wine, whereas in the good wine he found the yeast cells alone without any additional bacteria. He was thus able to demonstrate that wine will go sour if it contains organisms other than yeast.

In 1877 Pasteur published a book in which he showed that deterioration of beer also occurs if foreign bacteria are present. He described how, when he was invited to one of the large London breweries in 1871, he took his microscope with him, and in the presence of the managers, examined a sample of their yeast used to make porter. He decided that, since he saw other micro-organisms amongst the yeast cells, the porter was probably not satisfactory, and was pleased to find that the brewers did not disagree. He then studied the yeast used to make other types of beer and found them similarly contaminated. Next, he was asked to examine under the microscope one sample of beer which was cloudy and another which was clear, and quickly recognized a large number of bacteria in the cloudy sample, but also, after careful examination, found a few in the clear one. From this he concluded that both samples would rapidly spoil and were even then not at their best: to this everyone present had somewhat reluctantly to agree.

As bacteria could spoil wine and beer, it was obvious to Pasteur that it was essential to avoid introducing them during manufacture, or to kill them if already present. He realized that, even by the most careful technique of preparation, it would be impossible to avoid a few gaining entry, which would then multiply, so that the only practical method would be to kill any organisms after they had been introduced. He appreciated that this could be achieved by heat, but also knew that excessive heat would spoil the wine, so he tried the effect of adding various chemicals, but without success. He then developed a process of rapid heating to only about 55° C, out of contact with air, and found that this was sufficient to kill the bacteria, without spoiling the wine. This process soon became known throughout the world as pasteurization and has been used ever since for the preservation of wine, beer and milk.

Before the Renaissance, it was generally believed that plants and animals could, in certain circumstances, be created from any inanimate matter. This possibility is mentioned by several early writers, including Aristotle (384–322 B.C.), and as late as the sixteenth century Van Helmont (1577–1644), a celebrated chemist, reported that one could create mice at will by placing some dirty linen together with a piece of cheese in a container! In the seventeenth century it was still thought that plants and certain small creatures such as flies, ants, spiders and other insects were produced by abiogenesis. This was challenged by Francesco Redi (1626–97) who conducted experiments to show that this theory of spontaneous generation was untrue, at least for animals large enough to be seen with the naked eye. It remained however the general opinion that the living organisms of microscopic size found in large numbers in decaying organic material were produced by a chemical reaction and thus by a form of spontaneous generation. This theory was supported by the testimony of a Catholic priest, John Needham (1713–81), who stated that he had observed the spontaneous creation of living microscopic organisms, but it was refuted by the Italian anatomist, Spallanzani (1729–99) who conducted experiments to show that it was impossible.

It was well recognized that putrefaction in organic matter could be prevented by heating it to a high temperature, so that any microbes present would be killed; also that, provided it was then protected from the air, no further microbes would appear in it; but that if it was exposed to the air they would reappear. Those who believed that these microbes developed by spontaneous generation, inferred from these observations that this process would only occur in the presence of oxygen. Others realized that a more likely explanation was that the microbes were already present in the air and were deposited on the substance. This controversy raged fiercely until Louis Pasteur finally produced evidence to solve the problem. Several people tried to prove him wrong but, by his expert technique, with close attention to detail, they were eventually silenced. He not only solved this particular dispute but, in the course of his experiments, established proper methods of working with micro-organisms which had not been adopted previously.

He first demonstrated the presence of bacteria in the air by drawing air through a tube plugged by a cotton-wool filter. The dust which collected in this filter was then examined and found to contain numerous microscopic organisms. When this dust was sprinkled on to an organic substance, previously heated to kill off bacteria in it, and kept in a vacuum, there was a rapid growth of micro-organisms. There could therefore be no doubt that these micro-organisms had been present in the dust from the air, and it has since been shown that air is in fact an important carrier of bacteria harmful to man.

One of the experiments which Pasteur conducted on this subject will remain a classic for all time. He took a number of flasks filled with a liquid containing yeast and sugar, drew out the neck of each flask to a fine point by heating it in a flame, and then boiled the liquid to drive out the air and destroy anything living in it. The flasks were then sealed off completely by heating the drawn-out ends with a blowpipe. They were now free of living material and, because of this, remained sterile for as long as they were kept sealed. He placed them in widely differing types of geographical location, and then broke the neck of each with a long pair of pincers so as to allow the introduction of air. This had to be done with the utmost care and attention to detail: the neck of the flask and the pincers had first to be heated to kill all bacteria on them, and he had to be careful to break the glass with the pincers held well above his head so that the air was not contaminated with dust from his clothes. Once the neck of a flask was broken the surrounding air surged in to fill the vacuum already created, and each flask was then resealed in a flame. Some of them remained sterile while others developed a profuse growth of bacteria. He showed from these experiments that bacteria were either absent or few in number in the high mountainous districts, but plentiful in low-lying ground. At the same time he was able to produce irrefutable proof that microbes will not appear in an organic substance when it is exposed to air, unless they are already present in the air. It is important to note that Pasteur took great care to see that there was no contamination of the flasks to spoil his experiment, and that he achieved this by sterilizing the instruments and apparatus by heat—a method which has been adopted by bacteriologists ever since. The arguments about the possibility of spontaneous generation would never have raged so fiercely or for so long, if other workers in his day had been as careful. It should be mentioned that the English physicist, John Tyndall, also deserves credit for helping to lay the ghost of spontaneous generation by his experiments, of which accounts were published in 1876 and 1877 and, together with some other lectures, in a book entitled *Essays on the floating matter of the air in relation to putrefaction and infection*, issued in 1881. These experiments confirmed Pasteur's findings in every way.

Another of Pasteur's important investigations was into diseases which affect silkworms. The knowledge gained about the behaviour of disease-producing bacteria and the control of epidemics in these insects, was to prove extremely useful to him when he later studied the part played by micro-organisms in diseases which affect man. It may be recalled that, by a strange coincidence, it had also been work on silkworms that led the Italian, Agostino Bassi (1773–1856) to confirm for the first time that disease can be caused by living micro-organisms. Now, in the middle of the nineteenth century, just about the time of Bassi's death, silkworms were again decimated by disease to such an extent that the industry in France was on the verge of ruin, and the epidemic had spread to Italy, Spain and Austria, eventually affecting the industry in Greece, Turkey, China and Japan. Pasteur was asked by the French Minister of Agriculture to study the problem and began his investigation in 1865, knowing nothing of the habits of silkworms, and little about any micro-organisms which might infect them. He applied himself assiduously to the problem but it was five years before he reached a solution. The first two years of the study were marred by personal sorrow; in the first year his father died and this was followed later in the year by the death of his two-year-old daughter. The following year he was to suffer the loss of another daughter at the age of twelve from typhoid fever—a poignant reminder of the frequency with which parents had to face the death of children in the days before bacterial infections could be controlled.

During the course of the next three years, he was helped in the investigation by his wife and one surviving daughter, and eventually was able to show how certain diseases in silkworms could be avoided. It was time well spent because he was not only able to bring back prosperity to the industry in France but, perhaps of more importance, he acquired basic knowledge which was to prove of great value when he came to study disease in higher animals and man a few years later. He appreciated this himself, and advised those who came to help him in later years to read about his investigations into silkworms, as he believed this would give them a good introduction to this type of work.

Pasteur's work, including his studies into fermentation, his observations on the effect of micro-organisms in milk, beer and wine, and his epidemiological studies into diseases which affect silkworms, played an important part in leading doctors to consider the possibility that some diseases which affect human beings might also be brought about by microbes. This idea was not however readily accepted, as it seemed unreasonable to some people that disease in man could be brought about by minute living particles. It was accepted that microscopic organisms were found in diseased or dead tissue, but it was considered that they were more likely to be secondary invaders than the actual cause of the disease. Obermeier in 1868 reported that he had constantly found large numbers of spiral shaped organisms in blood of patients suffering from a disease called relapsing fever. It has in fact been confirmed since then that these particular microbes are the cause of this condition, but the discovery of organisms in the blood of a patient with a disease is not sufficient to prove that the disease is caused by the organisms, without further supporting evidence. Many people believed that, once the body became diseased, micro-organisms could appear in the affected tissue *de novo*, whilst others thought that tissues devitalized by disease were more prone to secondary invasion by micro-organisms entering the body from outside. It was therefore necessary, in order to prove that a disease was caused by certain specific organisms, for someone to show that, not only were they constantly present in this disease, but that they could be isolated and were then capable of reproducing the disease in another animal. The first man to supply such evidence was Robert Koch.

3

THE ENEMY NAMED

Robert Koch (1842–1910) showed an interest in science from an early age and, under the guidance of his father, became a proficient geologist, botanist and zoologist, so that gradually, during his early years, he acquired an extensive collection of minerals, plants and animals. On leaving school he entered the University of Göttingen to study medicine. He was an able student who made the most of every opportunity. At the same time he was extremely fortunate in his teachers. His professor of anatomy was Jacob Henle, the man who laid down important criteria which he insisted should be fulfilled before any specific organisms could be accepted as the cause of a given disease. He also came under the influence of the famous pathologist Krause and, as his assistant, gained useful experience, including a thorough knowledge of the technique of microscopy.

After qualification in 1866 he held junior posts in hospitals at Hanover and Hamburg and then entered general practice. His career was interrupted by the Franco-Prussian war in which he served as an army surgeon. When this was over, he found he could not settle down again to the life of a general practitioner, so studied for a higher examination in medicine, which he passed in 1872. After this he worked as a physician at Wollstein in East Prussia, where he soon built up a busy and lucrative consultant practice. He bought expensive apparatus, including a microscope and equipment to carry out photomicrography, which he installed in a laboratory next door to his consulting room. During the next four years, in addition to his clinical work, he made a special study of the disease called anthrax which was particularly prevalent amongst both animals and man in his community. Repeated examinations of the blood and tissues of affected animals showed the presence of a certain type of bacterium which he managed to isolate and study outside the body. He was then able to inject the organism into mice, guinea-pigs and rabbits, and to produce a similar disease in them. This was the first time that an organism isolated from damaged tissue had been cultured in the laboratory and then used to infect another animal. It was an important landmark in the history of bacteriology, and the work was accepted by everybody, except a Frenchman called Paul Bert (1833–86) who conducted experiments designed to show that Koch's conclusions were wrong. The challenge was taken up by Louis Pasteur who hastened to the assistance of Koch, and who, by well designed and meticulously executed experiments, was able to support him in his views. It was from the evidence thus produced by Koch and Pasteur that the germ theory of disease became universally accepted.

It was now essential to study the characteristics of the various types of micro-organisms so that they could be separately named and divided into groups. German bacteriologists had made many limited attempts to do this but the first reasonably accurate and worthwhile classification was made by Ferdinand Cohn in 1872. He was handicapped however by a lack of knowledge of techniques for staining bacteria; these were later developed by Robert Koch and enabled him to make some of the most important contributions to this subject. Simple dyes had been used to stain bacteria for some time, but Koch was the first man to use the newly discovered aniline dyes for this purpose. These are very powerful and he found they readily adhered to bacteria, making them stand out prominently under the microscope. He also developed a method of photomicrography which helped him considerably in this work.

In 1880 Koch was appointed to work in the laboratories at Bonn University where, with the help of enthusiastic assistants, he soon published important advances in bacteriological technique. In order to study bacteria in the laboratory they must be cultured on special nutrient substances. Up to that time fluids such as broth or blood serum had been commonly used, but Koch found it was possible—and advantageous—to use solid media which included agar, a substance derived from the stems of various seaweeds found in Japan; he also used agar enriched with blood, gelatine and solidified blood serum. These substances remain in common use today together with others introduced since that time. It was by the use of such solid culture media that he was able to establish a very important method of separating bacteria so that a pure growth of each type could be obtained. As this method is still employed in routine laboratory work it will be described in detail.

A piece of wire bent to form a loop at one end is first heated to kill any bacteria adherent to it and a loop full of the specimen under examination is smeared over the surface of the culture medium which is then placed in an incubator to be kept warm at body temperature, 37° C, for about two days. At the end of this time it is found that different types of bacteria will have grown in individual clumps or colonies. A colony of each particular type has its own characteristic appearance so that a loop full of any one can then be transferred to a separate culture plate, and in this way a pure growth of each variety of bacteria present may be obtained. This simple and effective technique was a great advance, because up to that time accurate classification, with identification and naming of the particular organisms which cause different types of disease, had been seriously handicapped by inability to separate them. After this, progress was rapid and, by about the beginning of this century, scientists had identified and named most of the bacteria harmful to man.

Koch and his pupils were responsible for much of this work and he himself acquired much fame in 1882 by his discovery of the tubercle bacillus, the germ which causes tuberculosis. Most organisms grown on a culture medium produce visible colonies after incubation for about 48 hours but tubercle bacilli divide much more slowly and it is to Koch's credit that, instead of discarding his culture plates after a few days, he persevered and showed that visible colonies of these organisms could be produced after several weeks' incubation. It was from such a culture that he was able to produce tuberculosis in a number of susceptible animals.

His anatomy teacher Henle had stated in 1840 that 'before microscopic forms can be regarded as the cause of contagion in man they must be found constantly in the contagious material, they must be isolated from it and their strength tested'. Koch was able to fulfil all these criteria with the tubercle bacillus, and in an address before the International Medical Congress in Berlin in 1890 laid down even more exacting principles, now known as 'Koch's postulates', to which each different type of organism must conform before it may be regarded as the cause of a disease. First, the organism must be found in every case of the disease and under conditions which explain the pathological changes and clinical symptoms; secondly, it must not be found as an accidental organism in other diseases; thirdly, after it has been isolated from the body and cultivated in pure culture, it must have the ability to produce the disease in animals. These basic rules are given in detail to show the remarkable clarity of his approach to this subject. By his insistence on such strict criteria he dissuaded bacteriologists from too readily drawing unwarranted conclusions from their observations, but at the same time, by removing confusion, it led them to make rapid progress in the accurate identification of disease-producing organisms. It has not always proved possible to fulfil every one of Koch's postulates, but, by adhering to them as closely as possible, serious errors have been prevented. As he himself said 'as soon as the right method is found discoveries come as easily as ripe apples fall from the tree'.

After five years in Bonn he became professor of hygiene in the University of Berlin where he organized the first systematic student course in bacteriology ever to be given. A few years later, in 1891, he became Director of the Institute of Infectious Diseases in Berlin, an establishment which was built specially for him, under his direction.

In 1890 Koch reported the preparation of tuberculin which is a protein derivative of the tubercle bacillus. There is little doubt that, from the results he obtained with experiments on guinea-pigs, he thought it was possible to treat tuberculosis with this substance. Soon the news spread, by means of the public press, that Koch had found an effective treatment for this disease, and his laboratory in Berlin was immediately besieged by physicians and their patients. Tragedy and disillusionment were to follow, as none of them recovered but many were made worse. This was sad, not only for the patients and their families, but it was also a bitter disappointment for Koch who had up to then achieved so much success. His discovery of tuberculin however was not in vain, as its use in a certain test employed for the diagnosis of this condition subsequently proved of great value.

In 1904 he resigned from the Institute, and devoted the last six years of his life to travel and to the investigation of infectious diseases in the Tropics. Due to his development of appropriate methods most of the important micro-organisms had been thoroughly studied by the turn of the century and bacteriology had become a science in its own right.

Micro-organisms occur everywhere, and may be found in soil, water and air, as well as in plants, animals and man. There are an enormous number of different types: most of them are harmless to man; some are helpful and are used in industry as mentioned in the chapter about Pasteur, and only a few are harmful. They include bacteria, fungi and a group of allied organisms called actinomyces about which you will read more in a later chapter. In addition there are groups of higher organisms which include yeasts and protozoa.

Bacteria are distinguished from unicellular plant life by not containing chlorophyll and not having demonstrable nuclei. They are divided into cocci, bacilli, vibrios and spirochaetes. Cocci are spherical bodies and common examples which affect man include staphylococci, streptococci, pneumococci, gonococci and meningococci. Staphylococci are to be found in boils, carbuncles, abscesses and occasionally in a serious form of pneumonia. Streptococci cause such diseases as tonsillitis, erysipelas, cellulitis and childbirth or puerperal fever. Pneumococci cause one form of pneumonia. Gonococci are the cause of gonorrhoea, and meningococci give rise to one variety of meningitis. Bacilli are straight rod-shaped organisms, many of which move about with the help of one or more flagella; common examples of bacilli which are pathogenic to man include those responsible for diphtheria, typhoid fever, dysentery, tuberculosis, leprosy, anthrax, tetanus and gas gangrene. Vibrios consist of small actively motile organisms in the shape of a comma, of which a good example is the one which causes cholera. Spirochaetes are thin spiral quickly moving filaments; examples include the variety responsible for syphilis and the one which causes relapsing fever.

The fungi (moulds) consist of tubular branched filaments; two well-known diseases caused by such organisms are ringworm and thrush. The actinomyces are also made up of branched filaments but they have certain characteristics which distinguish them from true fungi; one of the most important diseases produced by a member of this group is actinomycosis. Protozoa are unicellular organisms but, unlike bacteria, their protoplasm is separated into cytoplasm and nucleus; malaria and amoebic dysentery are caused by protozoa.

Finally, there is the group of organisms called viruses which are so small that they cannot be seen under the magnification of an ordinary microscope. Some of the virus diseases which affect man include the common cold, influenza, measles, mumps, chicken-pox, smallpox and poliomyelitis. It was because bacteria form only a part of microscopic life that Sedillot, a surgeon, in 1878 introduced the term 'microbe' in the course of a discussion in the Paris Academy of Medicine, to describe any living organism so small as only to be visible under a microscope. The term has not become popular among scientists. Pasteur also considered that the term bacteriology was too limited and suggested that the science should be called microbiology.

After the science of microbiology had been established, it was possible to begin a systematic search for methods to combat the various germs responsible for disease. This has not proved a simple task, but much progress has been made over the past fifty years, often when least expected and at times almost as if by chance.

It was not by chance, however, but through the pioneer work of Louis Pasteur, that the English surgeon Lister was able to develop a technique whereby the body could be opened and extensive operations performed without wounds becoming infected with bacteria from the surrounding air and from the hands and instruments of the surgeons. Hospital wards in his day were full of the stench of uncontrolled sepsis and patients' wounds dripped with pus, became gangrenous, and often gave rise to an overwhelming blood poisoning. Patients who came into hospital without much infection soon developed it once admitted and it was a frequent occurrence for the dreaded streptococcal infection called erysipelas to sweep through a hospital ward. The patients in those days had little chance to leave hospital alive; they might survive the hazards of extensive surgical procedures, but the possibility of withstanding attack by the countless bacteria present in the atmosphere of a hospital ward at that time was slight.

Joseph Lister, son of a London wine merchant, was professor of surgery in Edinburgh when he read how Louis Pasteur had shown that micro-organisms were responsible for the putrefaction of organic material and that different types of these bacteria were widely distributed in the atmosphere. He was much impressed by Pasteur's emphasis on the possible significance of this finding with regard to the spread of disease. Although Pasteur himself was not in a position to carry out experiments to prove it, Lister was convinced that infection in surgical wounds must be produced by germs from outside the body and searched for some chemical to destroy those found in the air, on surgical instruments and on surgeons' hands. He selected for his purpose carbolic acid which had first been prepared by a Manchester chemist named Calvert and which had already been used to deodorize and to disinfect sewage at Carlisle. He applied a dilute solution to all wounds and insisted that everything touching the wound, including the surgeons' hands, his instruments and dressings, must all be immersed in it.

Lister first used his antiseptic technique in March 1865, when he operated on a patient suffering from a compound fracture of the leg, and in 1867 published the results of treating such cases by this method. It was previously accepted that most patients with broken bones exposed to the air on account of extensive wounds, became seriously ill from infection, with the tissues covered in pus, so that it was often necessary to perform mutilating amputations, from which the patients frequently died. Lister however was able to report that out of eleven cases, who before this time would have certainly followed this course, nine recovered successfully, one had to undergo an amputation and only one died. This was a remarkable achievement and one of the most important landmarks in the history of surgery. A year later he wrote a further article 'On the Antiseptic System of Treatment in Surgery'. He was fully conscious of his debt to Pasteur, who first inspired him to take up this work, and often publicly acknowledged this fact. In 1874 he wrote a letter to Pasteur in which he said 'Allow me to take this opportunity to tender you my most cordial thanks for having by your brilliant researches demonstrated to me the truth of the germ theory of putrefaction and thus furnished me with the principle upon which the antiseptic system could be carried out. Should you at any time visit Edinburgh, it would, I believe, give you sincere gratification to see at our hospital how largely mankind is being benefited by your labours.'

In spite of these outstanding results his ideas were not readily accepted and he had to face much criticism from sceptics both in this country and in other parts of the world. In 1877, he decided to give up his post of professor of surgery at Edinburgh, where he had been from 1869, to take an appointment at King's College Hospital, London. His Scottish students, unwilling to lose a successful and popular teacher, signed a petition asking him to reconsider his decision. He realized, however, that his method of antiseptic surgery was gaining acceptance and being applied daily in many parts of the world, but not in London, so he considered it was his duty to work there in order to show that surgery would never be safe until his technique was adopted. Thus he left his friends in Edinburgh, gave up a large private practice and started afresh at the age of fifty in a new and hostile environment. His London colleagues showed cold disinterest in his methods and openly snubbed him in front of students who in turn adopted an apathetic attitude and ignored him. Also the nurses, who had been working with eminent men of that day and who naturally enough had implicit faith in their methods, were rebellious and made no effort to hide their disapproval of his technique. But his results continued to be so outstanding that, after a short time, his critics were silenced and his method universally adopted. In recognition of his achievements he received the Order of Merit in 1902. He lived long enough to see how greatly his antiseptic method improved surgery all over the world before he died, in 1912, at the age of eighty-five. Many people wrote about his personality and his achievements but perhaps their sentiments were most aptly summed up in the report of the Royal College of Surgeons which said, 'His gentle nature, imperturbable temper, resolute will, indifference to ridicule and tolerance of hostile criticism, contrived to make him one of the noblest of men. His work will last for all time. Humanity will bless him for evermore and his fame will be immortal.'

4

DEFENCE MEASURES

It has long been recognized that there are certain diseases which, if survived, never attack the victim again. The Greek historian, Thucydides (464–404 B.C.), wrote that when plague was raging in Athens during the Peloponnesian wars the sick and dying would not have received attention had it not been for the devotion of those who had already suffered from it and who knew that they could not therefore catch it a second time. It was also well known in Ancient China that an adult, pock-marked from an attack of smallpox as a child, did not develop it again when exposed in an epidemic. It therefore soon became apparent that, once a person had overcome certain infections, a change took place in his body with the development of some defence mechanism which protected him from further attacks. Further, it was quickly recognized that this protective change inside the body could occur as a result of only a mild attack of the disease. The Chinese found that powder made from the dry crusts taken from a case of smallpox sniffed up the nose produced an attack of the disease, sufficiently mild not to be dangerous, but which at the same time gave protection from further attacks.

Smallpox was brought to Europe, from the Orient, by the Crusaders in the twelfth century. By the seventeenth century it had become widespread in Britain, with severe epidemics, in which one out of every four people infected died and many survivors were blinded and others grossly disfigured by the marks left by the pox. In 1717 Lady Mary Wortley Montagu, wife of the British Ambassador in Turkey, introduced inoculation into this country. The method used at that time was to induce a mild form of the disease, by drawing a thread, soaked in fluid from a smallpox pustule, through a small incision made into the arm. At first it was tried out on six condemned prisoners, and after it had been shown to be successful with them, several members of the royal household were inoculated. Following this, it became an established practice, and people clamoured to have the disease artificially induced. The Quaker physician, Thomas Dimsdale (1712–1800), practised it widely, and became so famous that news of him reached the Empress Catherine of Russia who summoned him to St Petersburg to inoculate herself and her son. He was fearful lest something might go wrong and planned how he would escape should any disaster occur; he must have felt very relieved when he was able to write in his diary 'She has had the smallpox in the most desirable manner which now thank God is over!' He had good cause for anxiety because the disease produced in this way although usually mild was not always so; also, it was as contagious as the naturally occurring disease and required the isolation of the patient for a number of weeks.

As there were these serious disadvantages, people were only too willing to abandon this method of immunization as soon as a better one was found. It had been a popular belief for some time amongst country folk that a person infected from cows with a mild variety of pox was protected from the far more serious condition of smallpox. This was brought to the notice of the Gloucestershire medical practitioner, Edward Jenner (1749–1823), when he diagnosed smallpox in a dairymaid, who immediately told him that this was impossible as she had already suffered from cowpox. He decided to make some observations about this for himself and closely studied the effect of smallpox inoculation in patients already known to have had cowpox. He found that the reaction around the incision, in such patients, was negligible and there was no general constitutional disturbance. This convinced him that the dairymaid was right about cowpox giving protection against smallpox. In May 1796 he induced cowpox in an eight-year-old boy by the insertion of some fluid into his arm, obtained from blisters on the hand of a young woman suffering from this disease. Next, he inoculated him with fluid taken from a case of smallpox and no reaction occurred. Thus, for the first time, a person had been protected from smallpox by the artificial introduction of the milder form of pox which normally affects cows. It was for this reason that this preventive technique became known as vaccination, from the Latin word *vacca*—a cow.

As with all new and revolutionary ideas, there was much criticism and scepticism about the method, so that Jenner received strong opposition from many of his colleagues, particularly as, at that time, it was not free from complications. Occasionally, it led to bad ulcers developing at the site of inoculation and, in addition, some patients developed smallpox in spite of having been vaccinated. Nevertheless, it was soon realized that the benefits far outweighed any of these disadvantages and the method was widely practised. Jenner became famous and his country rewarded him for his outstanding contribution to medical science by a parliamentary grant of £10,000 in 1802 and a further £20,000 in 1806.

Knowledge of his technique soon spread abroad, and the success of vaccination against smallpox encouraged people to develop similar methods of preventive inoculation against other diseases prevalent at that time. A Frenchman, Auzias-Turenne, believed that it might be possible to prevent the ravages of syphilis by inoculation with a mild form of the disease and went so far as to advocate to the Paris Academy of Medicine that this should be performed on all the youth of France! He also believed that it would prove possible to develop methods to protect people against other diseases, such as anthrax, cholera and rabies; although he himself was not able to achieve this, he attained a good theoretical understanding of the subject, as is shown in his book entitled *La Syphilisation*, published in 1878. It is obvious that his ideas were closely studied by medical research workers at that time, and it is said that Louis Pasteur, who had developed a particular interest in this subject as a result of being much impressed by Jenner's work on smallpox vaccination, often read and made copious notes from the book, determined to find similar methods to apply to other diseases. An accident which occurred about a year after the book was published gave Pasteur his first important lead. In the spring of 1879 he began to study cholera in chickens. Towards the end of the summer, he took some chicken cholera bacteria from an old culture which had been in the laboratory for some months and injected them into healthy chickens, in the hope of inducing the disease. He was not successful. Therefore, he obtained a fresh supply of bacteria, from chickens already suffering from the disease, and when these were injected into healthy chickens, they readily induced the illness. Next, he injected these virulent organisms into chickens which had already been given bacteria from the old culture and once again he failed to produce any ill effects. Pasteur, with his great ability for accurate deduction, realized what must have happened. The chicken cholera bacteria kept in his laboratory all through the summer had lost most of their virulence and power to produce disease but, when injected into chickens, they still had the ability to bring about changes which made the chickens immune to further attack by virulent organisms. He had thus stumbled upon another disease against which artificial immunity could be induced. In order to show that the process was somewhat akin to Jenner's use of cowpox, he referred to this also as vaccination and the term has subsequently been used for many other types of immunization. This observation with chickens was of fundamental importance as it led him and others to work out similar methods of vaccination against other infections, so that today there are highly effective methods of immunization against a wide variety of diseases.

He discovered that to make disease-producing bacteria lose their virulence it was necessary to employ a different technique in each case. Within four years he had been successful with four conditions, of which two, anthrax and rabies, affect man. He studied anthrax because of observations he made on sheep affected with this disease. He had noticed that a flock of sheep grazing for a long time in a field where an animal which had died of anthrax had been buried, were not harmed when virulent anthrax bacilli were injected into them, whereas a similar injection into other sheep resulted in death. He deduced from this that the healthy sheep must have absorbed small amounts of anthrax bacteria from the dead animal and that this had brought about protective changes in their bodies, with the production of resistance to the disease. He therefore devised a method of growing anthrax bacteria in the laboratory by which they lost most of their virulence, and found that these attenuated organisms, on injection into animals, protected them from the effects of virulent bacteria. This was a very important observation because anthrax was prevalent in animals at that time and the cause of much financial loss to farmers. Many people however would not accept Pasteur's claims and his enemies, at the instigation of a veterinary surgeon named Rossignol, set out to ridicule him by staging a large-scale, much publicized experiment. Animals were taken to Rossignol's fields at Pouilly le Fort, near Melun, and a number vaccinated with Pasteur's attenuated bacilli and then inoculated some days later with virulent germs; at the same time, as a control, a similar number were inoculated with virulent germs alone. The vaccinated animals consisted of twenty-four sheep, one goat and six cows, and the controls consisted of twenty-four sheep, one goat and four cows. On 2 June 1881 a great crowd assembled to watch the result of the experiment. Pasteur approached the farm somewhat nervously, only to find however on arrival that all cynicism had disappeared and that everyone there was full of admiration and respect for him; the experiment had fully justified his claims. All the vaccinated sheep and cows were well; twenty-one of the control sheep were dead, two others died that morning in front of the crowd and the last one died at the end of the day. Also, the four control cows were ill. Obviously, with results like these, it was not long before anthrax immunization was widely practised with an enormous reduction in the death-rate amongst sheep.

A few months after his triumph at Pouilly le Fort, Pasteur attended the Medical Congress in London, where he suggested that when referring to the various methods of immunization which were being discovered the terms 'vaccine' and 'vaccination' should be used in all cases, in order to pay tribute to 'the merit and immense services rendered by one of the greatest men of England, your Jenner'.

Pasteur's interest in anthrax immunization obviously arose because his initial observations with sheep had suggested to him that immunization to this disease might be a possibility, and because the disease was widespread and affecting the nation's economy. His reason for wishing to develop a method of immunization against rabies was rather less obvious as it was not a disease which caused many deaths by comparison with other far more prevalent diseases, the causative germ had not been identified and, since it chiefly affected dogs and wolves, experiments were difficult and costly. It is, however, an extremely distressing and fatal disease which can affect anyone attacked by an infected animal. The other name for it, hydrophobia, literally translated means fear of water, because of the alarming convulsions a patient undergoes at the sight of water. These may be induced by offering the person a glass of water. As the glass touches the mouth, the head is thrown back in a series of spasmodic jerks, breathing becomes difficult and any water reaching the mouth is immediately ejected. These violent convulsions are brought about by painful spasms in the muscles which control swallowing and breathing and make the disease intensely frightening both for the sufferer and onlookers. It is said that Pasteur's interest in rabies was stimulated by vivid memories of the time when, during his childhood, an infected wolf attacked a number of men in his village. He watched while one of the victims had his bites cauterized with a red hot iron at a blacksmith's shop, in an attempt to prevent the development of the disease and later he learnt that many of them died after prolonged suffering.

As Pasteur knew that the causative organisms of rabies attacked the brain and spinal cord, he took spinal cords from rabbits which had died from the disease and suspended the cords in dry sterile air. He found that, as a result of this process, the rabies organisms in the nervous tissue lost their virulence and he could then use an emulsion of these cords as a vaccine. This vaccine was first used in dogs, was found to be effective and later saved many people from suffering. At first he had to face much bitter opposition and criticism from colleagues, who considered the method to be highly dangerous, but ultimately the discovery was to make him famous.

A person bitten by a rabid dog does not necessarily contract the disease; it depends on the number and character of the bites and on which part of the body they are inflicted. For the disease to develop, the germs have to travel from the bite to invade the central nervous system, and the time which elapses between the person being bitten and the development of symptoms is usually about one or two months. Pasteur suggested that advantage might be taken of this long interval, by vaccinating a person soon after he had been bitten, so that some immunity could be developed by the time the organism reached the brain and spinal cord. He carried out experiments by inoculating dogs bitten by rabid animals and the results appeared to be promising. It needed much courage however to take the next step and to inject the vaccine into a human being exposed to the disease for, not only might the patient not develop symptoms if left untreated, there was also a chance that the vaccine itself might cause trouble.

Pasteur was therefore very hesitant about using it, especially as well-informed medical opinion considered it to be an unwarranted risk, but he was forced to act when Joseph Meister, a boy aged nine, was brought to him from Alsace on 6 July 1885 suffering from bites on the hands, legs and thighs, from a rabid dog. Pasteur knew that the chances of the boy getting rabies from the bites were very high and felt he could not just stand by to watch this happen, so he gave him a course of injections, which to his great relief had no ill effects. The boy returned safely to Alsace. When this lad grew up he became a gatekeeper at the Pasteur Institute in Paris, where he died in 1940, for rather than let the German invaders force him to open the crypt where Pasteur was buried, he committed suicide.

The second case treated by Pasteur was that of Jean Baptiste Jupille, a fifteen-year-old shepherd, who saw a dog about to savage some children. He attacked it with his whip, but in so doing received numerous extensive bites. The dog was subsequently found to be suffering from rabies and the boy was rushed to Paris for treatment. He fortunately survived and his great bravery towards those children is commemorated in a statue which stands today in front of the Pasteur Institute.

These two dramatic recoveries were soon widely reported, so that before long, a large number of people bitten by dogs demanded vaccination from Pasteur. This method of treatment was much criticized by his colleagues, who argued that few people who are bitten develop the disease, and that the vaccine itself was equally dangerous. He had a certain number of failures, which were made much of by his opponents, but an English Commission, set up in 1888, to investigate the validity of his claims, expressed confidence in the value of his work in the following words: 'From the evidence of all these facts we think it is certain that the inoculations practised by M. Pasteur on persons bitten by rabid animals have prevented the occurrence of hydrophobia in a large proportion of those who, if they had not been so inoculated, would have died of the disease.' The Commission also recognized that by this technique he had established a new method which might be applicable against other diseases. 'We believe that the value of this discovery will be found much greater than can be estimated by its present utility for it shows that it may become possible to avert by inoculation even after infection other diseases besides hydrophobia.'

This was the real crux of the matter, for, although immunization against rabies may not have been more successful in reducing the number of deaths from the disease than have strict laws enforcing the muzzling of dogs, it was his work on rabies, anthrax and other diseases that established important basic principles. It showed that it is possible to reduce the virulence of organisms, so that, when injected into animals or man in this weakened state, they do not cause harm, but set up protective changes. Since that time, it has been possible to apply this to other diseases, including diphtheria, whooping cough, typhoid fever, tetanus, tuberculosis, yellow fever and, more recently, poliomyelitis.

5

CHEMICAL POISONS

The earlier chapters have shown that in the struggle against disease it was only possible to adopt commonsense general rules of hygiene until, with the discovery of the microscope, the enemy was identified. It was then possible to develop more accurate defence measures, including a technique to prevent the introduction of infection into wounds during surgical operations, and the stimulation of the natural defence mechanisms of the body by vaccination. The next step in the war against disease-producing bacteria would be to kill them in a direct manner with some chemical poison, but it was soon realized that this would present difficulties, as any poison which would kill bacteria was just as likely to damage the tissue cells of the body. A certain amount of encouragement, however, was derived from the fact that, during the course of centuries, a few chemical substances had accidentally been found to be effective against a small number of diseases.

As long ago as the sixteenth century the use of the metal antimony was advocated by that colourful character Paracelsus (1493–1541) whose real name, in keeping with his flamboyant personality, was Philippus Theophrastus Aureolus Bombastus von Hohenheim. He styled himself Paracelsus because, with his singular lack of humility, he wished to be identified with Celsus, the celebrated Roman medical author, whose eight famous books, entitled *De re Medicina*, were written about A.D. 30. Paracelsus has been accused of many hard things: charlatanism, drunkenness and boastfulness; some said he was mad. Nevertheless, he was a prolific and provocative writer. One famous book which is now acknowledged to have been written by him had the somewhat strange title *The Triumphal Chariot of Antimony* (1604); in this, he recommended the medicament for a wide variety of maladies without offering much evidence upon which to base his faith in its efficacy. Since that time however it has proved to be of great value in the treatment of many tropical infections.

Paracelsus is also said to have introduced mercury in the treatment of syphilis; this was certainly sound practice, as time has confirmed its value in this disease and, in fact, it continued to be used long after certain arsenical compounds were discovered by Ehrlich at the beginning of this century.

Another microbial disease which has been successfully treated with a chemical substance for several centuries is malaria, the cause of much suffering and death in many parts of the world. A specific cure for it, introduced to Europe in the seventeenth century, was found in the bark of the cinchona tree which grows in South America. In Great Britain its use against malaria, a serious and prevalent disease at that time, was popularized by the famous physician Thomas Sydenham (1624–89). For a long time there was a romantic legend that cinchona bark was first brought to Europe by Lady Ana de Osorino, Countess of Chinchon, the wife of the Viceroy of Peru. It was said that when she was in Lima, early in the seventeenth century, she developed malaria, and at the suggestion of a local governor, took some powder prepared from the bark of the tree, and was miraculously cured. In gratitude for this, she distributed large quantities of the powder to the citizens of Lima, and later introduced it into Spain. Unfortunately the story is not true, because A. W. Haggis, writing in the *Bulletin of the History of Medicine* in 1941, states that he has studied the diary of the Countess and found that she died in Spain before her husband was ever sent to Peru, and that his second wife, who did go to Peru with him, not only was never ill there, but died on the return journey before she reached home. It would seem that the truth is that the bark was introduced into Europe from South America by Jesuit missionaries and priests.

At the beginning of the nineteenth century, the German Sertürner, extracted morphine from opium in poppies. This stimulated two young French chemists, Pelletier and Caventou, to attempt to separate active ingredients from other plants. From a South American plant, called ipecacuanha, they extracted emetine which has since been found to have a specific action against the parasite responsible for amoebic dysentery. Later, by a similar method, they separated the active principles in cinchona bark and, when they reported this discovery in 1820, called the part which cured malaria quinine, a name derived from the old Peruvian word for the cinchona tree, quina-quina.

About this time, on account of the world demand for this drug, which only came from trees in South America, certain nations with Eastern dependencies where malaria was rife, particularly the British and the Dutch, became alarmed in case the supply should be insufficient for their needs. The British therefore transferred seeds and plants to India and Ceylon, and the Dutch to Java. At first the British seemed to be more successful, as their plantations in India grew hardy trees (*Cinchona succi rubra*) but it was found that this particular species gave a poor yield of quinine. The Dutch, on the other hand, had the good fortune to buy, by chance, a small quantity of seeds from an Englishman, Charles Ledger, who had lived in Peru for a long time; it turned out that the trees from these seeds (later called *Cinchona ledgerina*) gave an exceptionally high yield of quinine, but unfortunately proved very difficult to rear. The Dutch overcame this difficulty by grafting them on to robust trees of the *Cinchona succi rubra* variety, and by this means established trees in Java, as hardy as the British ones in India, but giving a very much greater yield of quinine.

Mercury against syphilis and quinine against malaria were therefore two of the earliest examples of chemical substances which, when taken into the body, killed disease-producing micro-organisms. They were first used long before the specific micro-organisms had been identified, as it was not until 1880 that Alphonse Laveran, a young medical officer in the French army stationed in Algeria, first demonstrated the malarial parasite in the red cells of patients, nor until 1905, that Fritz Schaudinn, in Germany, identified the organism responsible for syphilis.

The identification of bacteria under the microscope towards the end of the last century stimulated the German chemist, Paul Ehrlich, to search systematically for chemical substances which, when taken into the body, would kill harmful bacteria, while doing as little damage as possible to the tissue cells. It was about this time that aniline dyes were first manufactured and found to be not only of great value in the textile industry but also in the newly developed science of microscopy, as they stained tissue cells and bacterial cells vivid colours, thus allowing a detailed examination of them to be made under the microscope. It was noticed that these dyes were absorbed by different types of cells in a highly selective manner so that each type stood out in its own distinctive colour. This observation led Ehrlich to consider whether he could find a dye which would specifically adhere to bacteria in the body, and thus kill them, but which, at the same time, would not affect other cells. The development of this idea led him eventually to discover important anti-bacterial drugs, and, by the adoption of a similar approach, his pupil, Gerard Domagk, discovered further ones of great value after the First World War.

Paul Ehrlich was the first man to place the search for antibacterial chemical substances on a scientific basis and it was he who introduced the term 'chemotherapy' for this type of treatment, the use of which has now been extended to include the killing of cancer cells by similar substances.

Derivatives of fungi have also been found to have a highly poisonous effect on bacteria. The two most widely used, and best known, are penicillin and streptomycin, and they, with several others, belong to a group of drugs which are now called antibiotics.

It is a commonplace observation that certain animals help man by killing others that may be harmful to him but it is less well known that this also occurs in life visible only through the microscope. This phenomenon is readily demonstrated by a study of the micro-organisms in the soil. Animals excrete a large number of bacteria into the soil and infected animals are also buried there but, in spite of this, it is not the source of much disease. This is because organisms deposited in it are quickly killed, partly by the action of the sun, but also by other microbes which live there. It was an appreciation of this which led Selman Waksman to discover streptomycin. In addressing the National Academy of Sciences in Washington, in 1940, he said 'Bacteria pathogenic for man and animals find their way to the soil, either in the excreta of the hosts or in their remains. If one considers the period for which animals and plants have existed on this planet and the great number of disease-producing microbes that must have thus gained entrance into the soil, one can only wonder that the soil harbours so few bacteria capable of causing

1*a* Thirteenth-century leper colony (Paul La Croix: *Science et lettres au Moyen-Age*)

1*b* Jacob's Island, Bermondsey, when the stream was the sole water-supply and means of sewage disposal (Wellcome Historical Medical Museum)

2 Antony van Leeuwenhoek, a portrait by Verkolje (Rijksmuseum, Amsterdam)

3 Leeuwenhoek's "Microscope" (from C. Dobell: *Antony van Leeuwenhoek and His 'Little Animals'*, Dover Publications Inc., New York)

4a   Edward Jenner vaccinating a child with matter from the hand of Sarah Nelmes, who had contracted cowpox in milking (Bettmann Archive, New York)

4b   Pasteur supervising anti-rabic injection of patients bitten by mad animals (Bettman Archive, New York)

5*a* Lister carbolic steam spray
(Wellcome Historical
Medical Museum)

5*b* The first photographic
record of the phenome-
non of antibiosis (the
destruction of one micro-
organism by another).
Published in 1889 by
Doehle in a thesis at Kiel.
(Thesis now in the
Bodleian Library, Oxford.)
Anthrax bacilli were
grown over the entire
surface of the culture
medium. An organism
named by Doehle the
'Micro-coccus antraco-
toxicus' was planted in the
form of a square (*b*). This
inhibited the growth of the
anthrax bacilli within and
around the square (*c*) but
had no effect on the
anthrax bacilli growing
at the periphery (*a*)

6a Paul Ehrlich and Sahachiro Hata
(Wellcome Historical Medical Museum)

6b Gerard Domagk (*Münchener
Medizinisher Wochenschrift*,
J. F. Lehmanns Verlag,
Munich, 1953)

7a Sir Alexander Fleming and Sir Almroth Wright (Copyright *Illustrated*, reproduced in A. Maurois: *The Life of Sir Alexander Fleming*, Cape, London)

7b Plate culture of *Staphylococcus pyogenes*, incorporating tests of sensitivity to three antibiotics. It is resistant to the penicillin (top) but not to the streptomycin or tetracycline (L.P. Garrod and E.F. Scowen, *British Medical Bulletin*, **16** (1960), 23)

8*a* Sir Howard Florey

8*b* Professor E. B. Chain

8*c* Professor S. A. Waksman

infectious diseases in man and in animals. The soil was searched for bacterial agents of infectious diseases until the conclusion was reached that these do not survive long in the soil. The cause of the disappearance of these disease-producing organisms in the soil is to be looked for among the soil-inhabiting microbes antagonistic to the pathogens and bringing about their rapid destruction in the soil.'

This observation suggested to him that it might be possible to use some of these microbes which kill bacteria in the soil, or suitable extracts from them, to kill bacteria causing diseases in the body. This proved highly successful and many important antibiotics derived from soil microbes, in addition to streptomycin, have been produced.

The word antibiosis was first used, in 1889, by the Frenchman, Vuillemin, who said 'when two living bodies are closely united and one of the two exercises a destructive action on a more or less extensive portion of the other then we can say that "antibiosis" exists'. After this its use was mainly confined to the activities of micro-organisms, but the term antibiotic was originally an adjective applied to any organism which had a lethal effect on other organisms. Its modern usage as a noun, when referring to substances such as penicillin and streptomycin, began in 1941, when Waksman employed it to describe any chemical substance extracted from a micro-organism which had the ability to kill other pathogenic microbes.

Although much progress in the conquest of disease has been achieved during this century by the skilful utilization of the lethal effects of certain microbes on others, it should be made clear that the possibility was first considered as long ago as 1877. At that time Louis Pasteur, with his colleague Joubert, observed that anthrax bacilli growing in urine were often killed when the specimen became contaminated by other organisms from the air. They also noticed that animals infected with anthrax bacilli often did not die from this disease if, at the same time, they were also infected by other organisms. These observations led Pasteur to prophesy that, 'the time may come when we may utilise harmless microbes for combating harmful ones'.

Cantani, in 1885, had the original and ingenious idea, based on this principle, that micro-organisms might be used to attack harmful bacteria in the lungs. He attempted this by trying to kill the bacilli causing pulmonary tuberculosis in a patient, by insufflating into the lungs large quantities of ill-defined harmless organisms. This was the first time micro-organisms had been introduced into a patient's body in an effort to kill disease-producing bacteria.

In the laboratory similar efforts were made to inhibit the growth of organisms on culture plates by the action of others. A Swiss, Garré, in 1887 published work on this and in 1904 W. D. Frost, in Great Britain, described several methods for investigating the antagonistic properties of bacteria. Frost grew one type of bacteria in a liquid medium in a flask and another in a medium contained in a collodian sac suspended in the flask. He found that a substance which today would be called an antibiotic, produced by the bacteria in one medium, could diffuse through the collodian membrane and inhibit the growth of bacteria in the other.

In 1887, Emmerich, in Germany, showed that some protection could be given to rabbits suffering from experimental anthrax by the simultaneous injections of streptococci and in 1889, Bouchard, in France, reported that rabbits infected with this disease could be helped by the injection of organisms called pyocyaneus bacilli. Following this Emmerich and Low, ten years later, prepared an extract from these organisms called pyocyanase and found that, in the laboratory, this was capable of killing anthrax bacilli, typhoid bacilli, diphtheria bacilli, staphylococci and the causative organisms of plague. Therefore, they attempted to inject it into experimentally infected animals, but it proved too toxic and could only be used by local application. Thus, by the turn of the century, many attempts had been made to apply the principle of antibiosis and the successful extraction of pyocyanase gave promise that it might be possible to find similar, but more suitable, antibiotics in the future.

When Waksman began his search for antibiotic substances, in 1939, the first organism which he studied was once again the pyocyaneus bacillus, and its extract pyocyanase. Although pyocyanase, as before, did not prove very suitable as an antibiotic, its preparation helped him to develop a suitable technique for the extraction and purification of other substances from micro-organisms and allowed him to establish satisfactory methods for testing their properties.

The next group of microbes which he investigated was the actinomycetes (organisms of this group are also called 'Ray fungi' from their appearance under the microscope) and it was from these that, in 1943, he obtained streptomycin, the drug which was to play such a vital part in the control of tuberculosis, in addition to being useful against other infections.

He was not the first to work with actinomycetes. Much evidence had been produced long before this to show that these organisms, and extracts from them, had the power to kill other microbes. In 1917 Greig-Smith, in Australia, reported that he had noted that actinomycetes recovered from the soil had the power of stopping the growth of certain bacteria. Lieske, in 1921, published a monograph in German on *The Morphology and Biology of the Ray Fungi*, in which he discussed antibacterial chemical substances produced by the actinomycetes. Work on the same subject was published in French medical journals, by Gratia and Dath, in 1924 and 1925, and again by Gratia in 1934.

Similarly, Alexander Fleming's observations on the adverse effect of a mould on the growth of some staphylococci in 1928, which led to the discovery of penicillin, was not the first occasion on which a mould had been observed to have antibacterial properties. As long ago as 1896 Gosio described how he had obtained a crystalline substance from a mould of the penicillium family, which inhibited the growth of anthrax bacilli, and regretted that he was unable to perform animal experiments because of lack of material. Also, in 1913, Vaudremer published in a French medical journal an account of the effect of another mould, the *Aspergillus fumigatus*, which he found 'digested' the tubercle bacillus. As a result of this he carried out animal experiments, and injected filtrates of the mould into patients suffering from tuberculosis.

It may therefore be seen that the progress made in the twentieth century had its roots in the past. Further, it has to be realized that, even when this progress was made, final victory was not achieved easily, or quickly, but was dependent on the contributions of a large number of workers. For example, from the time that Fleming first made his original observation on the effect of a mould (subsequently identified as *Penicillium notatum*), it was another ten years before it achieved practical importance, when Florey, Chain and their team of workers at Oxford developed a technique which allowed them to produce an extract which was suitably purified for clinical use. Repeated attempts by various chemists before this had failed and it looked, at one time, as if the task might not be possible.

This chapter has outlined the evolution of ideas which led eventually to the discovery of important drugs for the treatment of microbial disease during this century. These discoveries had to wait until there were appropriate economic and social stimuli and until suitable progress has been made in the development of the ancillary sciences, but they could never have been achieved without the initial inspiration of pioneers. René Dubos in his book *Louis Pasteur* has a chapter devoted to the 'Mechanisms of Discovery' in which he says, 'because every discovery, even that which appears to first sight the most original and intuitive can always be shown to have roots deep in the past, certain students of the history of science believe that the role of the individual in the advancement of knowledge is in reality very small'. It is certainly true that any great discovery which is made by a research worker often depends on the valuable work of others in the past as well as on the good fortune that he is working on a given problem at the right time in the right place. When therefore we praise the men who have made great discoveries we should also remember all the other workers, sometimes nameless and often long forgotten, who prepared the way. In the next chapters the discovery of present-day antibacterial drugs will be discussed, beginning with the work of Paul Ehrlich, the father of modern chemotherapy.

6

GUIDED MISSILES

Paul Ehrlich, the only son of an inn-keeper, was born at Strehlen, Upper Silesia, in March 1854. His grandfather had been a keen scientist and Paul resembled him in appearance and aptitude. His father was not a practical man and the successful running of their business was due to his mother's drive and ability. Paul showed his interest in chemistry at an early age so that by the time he was eight the chemists in his town were already making cough drops according to his prescription! At school he was always trying out new chemical experiments. Latin and mathematics pleased him but he found German composition to be extremely difficult. His inability to write a competent essay nearly failed him in his school-leaving examinations; fortunately he had done well enough in his other subjects to compensate for this weakness.

After leaving school, he went to Breslau University but was unhappy there and moved during his first term to the newly founded University of Strasbourg. He was fortunate in Strasbourg to be taught by Professor Waldeyer, an outstanding chemist, who took a great interest in young Ehrlich, and encouraged him to do original work while only a student. His main interest right from the start was in the new aniline dyes which were then being produced in a German chemical works and, on his own initiative, he explored various ways in which these could be used to stain cells so as to make it easier to study them under the microscope. He was to continue this study throughout his time at the university and was responsible for the development of techniques which made a considerable contribution to the science of microscopy. He did not allow it however to interfere with his other studies, and in his third term at the university passed his 'Physikum'—an examination which is held at German universities in chemistry, botany, zoology, physics, anatomy and physiology. After this, he continued his medical studies by returning to the university at Breslau. One day a physician from the town of

Wollstein in Silesia visited the university to show the professor his work on the anthrax bacillus. He was conducted through the various laboratories and while there saw a student working industriously at his bench, 'That is little Ehrlich, who is very good at staining but will never pass his examinations', he was told. This was the first introduction that the famous bacteriologist, Robert Koch, had to the student who was not only to pass his examinations but, in later years, was to work in close collaboration with him.

He completed his university training at Leipzig where he continued his studies with dyes, not only in the laboratory but also in the little inn where he lodged. Years later, when he became famous, the innkeeper's daughter wrote to him to remind him of the time when all the towels in the house were marked with dyes in every shade of red and blue. Even the billiard table itself had suffered in the same way, for he made his experiments on this as there was nowhere else suitable.

It was at Leipzig, in the year 1878, that he graduated at the age of twenty-four as a doctor of medicine. His thesis for this degree dealt with the use of aniline dyes to stain preparations of tissue cells so that they might be studied under the microscope. In this thesis, he clearly brought out the basic principle that every dye has an affinity for certain specific types of cell, so that the one becomes readily bound to the protoplasm of the other. This fundamental observation later led him to examine the dyes again in a search for chemicals which might kill the cells of bacteria in the body, whilst leaving the surrounding tissue cells unaffected. It will thus be seen that this initial work of Ehrlich's, done before he was qualified as a doctor, served as the guide which led him to create the science of chemotherapy.

It is somewhat alarming to discover that, with the passing of years, this important thesis became lost in the archives of the university at Leipzig and it was only after his death that his wife and his friend Professor Leonor Michaelis succeeded in tracing the original. He actually published the main theme of his dissertation in a journal in 1877, one year before his thesis was presented to the university. Miss Martha Marquardt, his secretary from 1902 until the time of his death, has in recent years found a copy of this journal in the British Museum.

After qualifying as a doctor, Ehrlich became a house physician to Professor von Frerichs at the Charité Hospital in Berlin. The Professor immediately recognized the great ability of this young man and encouraged him in his research work. Ehrlich continued to take a special interest in the application of dyes and developed methods of staining samples of blood so that the various cells in it could readily be identified under the microscope. He was the first man to show that the white cells could be separated by their staining reactions into three distinct types; an observation which has proved of great practical importance. He soon became famous for this alone and professors from other universities travelled far to watch him demonstrate his methods. They were not only very impressed by his skill, but amazed by the simplicity of his apparatus, which consisted of nothing more than an iron plate on a tripod over a gas jet, some slides and a few dyes.

While he was still a house physician, he married the nineteen-year-old daughter of an industrialist in Upper Silesia. She was to remain his devoted and understanding companion for the rest of his life. There must have been times when she wished she saw more of him, because like many great men, he became heavily committed with his work and so devoted to his research studies that it was difficult to persuade him to take even a short holiday. He drove himself hard and rarely stopped to take proper meals but seemed to exist by drinking large quantities of mineral waters and smoking countless cigars. His energy was boundless and he fired all those around him with similar enthusiasm. He would always find time to explain his theories to anyone who was interested and would illustrate these theories by drawing with chalk on furniture, doors, or even the listener himself. His words would be punctuated by the frequent use of characteristic interjections which later in life became almost proverbial. One of his favourite expressions was, 'You see: you understand.' This frequent interjection also figured in his dictation, so that his first secretary at times became so confused that she included it in the typescript, to produce very curiously worded documents. Finally, the effort of concentrating to take down only the essentials proved too much and she found herself quite unable to do the work and ran away.

In 1882 Ehrlich attended a meeting of the Physiological Society of

Berlin when Robert Koch announced his momentous discovery of the tubercle bacillus. Immediately the lecture was finished, Ehrlich rushed back to his laboratory at the Charité Hospital, to stain with dyes, specimens of sputum coughed up by tuberculous patients. As it was late at night he looked round hastily for somewhere to put the slides to dry: he noticed the iron stove was cold, as the fire had been out for some hours, so he quickly put the slides down on the top of this. The next morning when the cleaner arrived, she lit the fire as usual not noticing the slides. Ehrlich arrived soon after to examine his specimens and to his horror saw what had happened. He rushed forward in dismay and quickly snatched them up, but to his amazement, after suitable treatment he found that they were successfully stained and on examining them under a microscope, the tubercle bacilli were seen to stand out very clearly as masses of short red sticks heaped together in clumps. By this lucky accident, he stumbled upon the important truth that staining of tubercle bacilli is best accomplished by heating the dye.

Ehrlich immediately informed Koch of his discovery and this was the beginning of a friendship and successful partnership in various research projects. Koch paid tribute to the importance of Ehrlich's work on the staining of tubercle bacilli in an article published in 1883, in which he said, 'It was soon found that, with Ehrlich's method of staining, the recognition of tubercle bacilli could readily be made use of in diagnosis'.

Life was going smoothly for Ehrlich when his chief, Professor von Frerichs, suddenly died. Unfortunately his successor, Professor Gerhardt, and Ehrlich found themselves to be at cross purposes and the friendly happy atmosphere changed to one where there was persistent tension. His new chief demanded that he should carry out dull routine clinical duties and discouraged him from doing any original work. Ehrlich, who had a sensitive personality, felt his spirit to be crushed and through frustration, became physically and mentally exhausted. To add to his troubles, before long, he began to show signs that he had developed pulmonary tuberculosis. He therefore resigned his post at the hospital and with his wife, went to live in Egypt for a time. It would seem that his tuberculosis was in fact only mild, but that the psychological stress to which he had been submitted had been the cause of most of his symptoms. In some of his autobiographical notes about this unhappy incident, he wrote somewhat pathetically, yet very understandably, 'when I felt so miserable and forsaken during the time with Gerhardt, I often stood before the cupboard in which my collection of dyes was stored and said to myself, "These are my friends which will not desert me"'.

After two years abroad he recovered his health and returned to Berlin in 1889. He first set up in a private laboratory, but before long, Robert Koch, who by now had become Director of the Institute for Infectious Diseases, offered him a post there. Ehrlich was delighted and it was here that the next phase of his life began, during which he was to make a notable contribution to work which was being done at that time in the treatment of diphtheria.

The fact that a patient suffering from a contagious disease is feverish, weak, listless and without appetite suggested to early observers that, when bacteria attack a part of the body, they not only cause local damage but also liberate a poison which circulates throughout the body. Loeffler, who identified the diphtheria bacillus under the microscope, suspected that these organisms produced a poison in the blood, but it was Roux and Yersin, in 1886, who proved that such a toxic substance actually existed. They cultured diphtheria bacilli in broth, then filtered off the bacteria from the broth. This broth, on injection into animals, proved fatal, showing that it contained a toxic substance. This discovery alerted people to the possibility that other organisms might produce a similar poison but only two other bacteria have been found to behave in this way, one being the tetanus bacillus. In 1890, von Behring and Kitasato demonstrated the presence of toxin in a broth culture of tetanus bacilli by showing that broth in which these bacilli had been grown, after filtration, produced tetanus in animals susceptible to this condition.

The next important step was the appreciation that the body, as part of its defence mechanism, produced antitoxins to neutralize these toxins. Von Behring and Kitasato demonstrated that when toxin from tetanus bacilli was injected into a rabbit a change took place in the serum, with the production of a substance which had the effect of neutralizing the toxins. They were then able to show that a mixture of toxin and serum, from an animal infected with the disease, was innocuous on injection into other animals, because the antitoxin contained in the serum neutralized the toxin. Following this, they demonstrated that serum which contained antitoxin was capable of protecting an animal exposed to a lethal dose of toxin. In addition to this work on tetanus, in the same year, von Behring reported finding similar antitoxins in diphtheria. It was now obvious, therefore, that, if a large amount of the appropriate antitoxin could be produced, so that it could be injected in high concentration, it would be a valuable means of treating a patient who had an overwhelming toxaemia from diphtheria. It was at this stage that Ehrlich contributed to the problem. Von Behring found that he was not able to produce an antitoxin in high enough concentration to be effective. Ehrlich showed that he could do this by repeated injections of toxin into the blood of horses. He also devised a method by which the amount of antitoxin present could be accurately measured, and later, he established a central institute in Germany where all antitoxin used for treatment was standardized. For the first time therefore there was now an effective treatment for diphtheria. It was unfortunate for Ehrlich that his happiness about this achievement was marred by von Behring, who tried to take unfair advantage over him about certain financial arrangements associated with the production of this antitoxin. This led to the irrevocable breaking of their friendship in a spirit of enmity and bad feeling.

The method was not so successful in the treatment of tetanus: spores from tetanus bacilli lie about in the dirt and enter the body, often when the skin surface has only been broken by minor cuts or abrasions. This leads to an illness characterized by intensely painful spasms of muscles, but the giving of antitoxin at this stage is useless as the toxin will have already entered the body cells. It is valuable however to give antitoxin immediately after any open injury, as a prophylactic measure, because it will then be available to neutralize toxin liberated into the blood stream, should infection with tetanus have occurred.

Ehrlich continued to work at Robert Koch's Institute for Infectious Disease until 1896, when he was invited to take a government appointment as Director of the State Institute for the Investigation and Control of Sera, which was due to be opened in Steglitz, a suburb of Berlin. The main purpose of this establishment was to enable the Prussian government to establish a tight control over the production of anti-diphtheria serum and other newly found sera. Ehrlich was delighted with his post, as he knew he would have a free hand with the work there and it meant that his long felt ambition to become head of a medical research unit, had at last been fulfilled. The buildings, however, were primitive, his laboratory was a dilapidated disused bakehouse, and the money available to him for research was limited and strictly controlled by a niggardly state budget. His enthusiasm and drive were immense and, in spite of these limitations, he and his assistants carried out important experiments on the effect of various chemicals injected into animals.

His work was so successful and he published such a large number of original papers in the medical journals, that Dr Altoff, the Director of the Prussian Ministry of Educational and Medical Affairs, felt that every opportunity should be given to this brilliant young investigator. Therefore, he approached the Lord Mayor of Frankfurt for help in improving Ehrlich's working conditions. Between them they succeeded in bringing about the foundation of the Institute for Experimental Therapy, which was opened in 1899, with Ehrlich as Director. It is obvious that such an institute would never have been built had it not been for the fact that Ehrlich had already shown remarkable progress in the application of chemistry to medical treatment. From the day of starting in this new institute, he had sixteen more years of life left to him, during which he made most of his greatest discoveries. It was a large and imposing building in south Frankfurt, near the hospital, with well equipped laboratories, library and reading rooms. It was an ideal environment for Ehrlich to develop the ideas on which he had already started working in Koch's laboratory and at Steglitz. The main principle of these ideas was based on his so-called 'side-chain' theory which was that, whenever there is infection with bacteria, various antibodies appear in the blood as part of the natural defence mechanism and, because of a specific affinity, become anchored by a side chain to the invading organisms, thus rendering them harmless. These antibodies behave in other words, like modern guided missiles and, indeed, Ehrlich often referred to them as magic bullets. He felt that, just as these substances are made inside the body for this purpose, it should be possible to make similar ones in the laboratory which, on being taken into the body, would poison the cells of bacteria, while having little effect on the normal cells of the body. He realized that such chemicals would be bound to have some toxic effect on the tissue cells and that it would be necessary to produce many different derivatives of substances, by altering their basic molecular structure, until one was found which would have a poisonous effect on bacteria with only a minimal effect on normal cells. He once tried to explain this theory, which was to guide him in his search for suitable anti-bacterial substances, to two English professors, Sir Almroth Wright and William Bullock, while they were travelling back from some conference, on the night train from Berlin to Frankfurt. He became so excited and carried away by his denouncement of his critics and by the elucidation of his theories, that the guard threatened more than once to turn all three of them off the train! Ehrlich had not only worked himself up into a state of feverish excitement, but had had a similar effect on his friends, who could see that it might well prove possible that this man, by his zeal and great knowledge of chemistry, could bring about a revolution in medical treatment. This in fact he did with the help of a team of workers, who with infinite patience, made hundreds of different chemicals and tried them out on countless animals artificially infected with many different types of disease.

He was a determined and somewhat autocratic director who insisted that his juniors carried out their allotted tasks as planned by him. He would not tolerate opposition or wilful evasion of his instructions by his staff, and if a man did not agree with his methods he had to resign. Although a hard taskmaster who expected those around him to achieve the same high standard as he set himself, he is said to have been at the same time friendly, jovial and very approachable. He was very fond of music and derived much pleasure from listening to all the popular tunes of the day played for him by a man who stopped his barrel organ outside his laboratory window. In addition he was always most helpful, kind and generous to those in trouble. It is known that he gave large sums of money to many people in distress or difficulty; he always found it difficult to refuse help and because of this people attempted to take advantage of such a kindly and sensitive soul. There were many times when he was left short of money himself because of the frequent demands of other people.

It was in this happy atmosphere that Ehrlich and his team zealously devoted their time to finding bacterial poisons. He was guided in this by experience gained from some of his other work. His study of antibodies and antitoxins produced inside the body, had led him to believe that similar chemicals might be found outside the body, which on ingestion would kill bacteria. His work with dyes and his observation that each one had a specific affinity for certain tissues, led him to the idea that it might be from similar substances that he could find chemicals which would be specially attracted to bacterial cells and would thus act as 'magic bullets', in a similar way to the chemical antibodies manufactured in the body.

The first chemicals with which he experimented in his search for antibacterial substances were therefore dyes. These were prepared, under the direction of Dr Ludwig Benda, at the Cassella Chemical Works in Frankfurt, which later became the famous I.G. Farbenindustrie. Among the dyes first tested were Trypaflavine, and Trypan red. They were injected into animals which had been inoculated with a variety of different disease-producing organisms. It was found that they were particularly effective against the germs responsible for sleeping sickness. This is a serious and, without treatment, usually fatal disease which affects the natives of Africa. Trypan red, which was most potent experimentally, was therefore tried out in the tropics and found to be successful in the treatment of patients with this disease. It is of great interest that Ehrlich's particular approach to his search for chemotherapeutic substances led him to gain his first success with a disease which was a scourge to people thousands of miles from his own land.

His second success, and the great triumph of his life, was when he discovered a chemical which killed the organisms responsible for syphilis. Syphilis had been a world-wide problem for many centuries. It was well recognized that it was a disease contracted during sexual intercourse which started with a small ulcer, usually on the genitalia, and that the infection spread from there to affect many organs of the body, including the brain and heart, so that the patient could ultimately become blind, paralysed, mad, or die from heart failure. In view of the serious consequences of this disease many remedies had been devised throughout the ages but the only one which had been found to have any real effect was mercury rubbed into the skin. This proved however to be of limited value and to have side effects which at times were almost as bad as the disease. The widespread enthusiasm which greeted Ehrlich's triumph when he at last gave the world a drug which was effective as well as safe, needs little imagination. It was not however found by chance, but by tedious, dogged and persistent systematic trial of hundreds of chemical substances used on thousands of animals.

Ehrlich himself was fond of saying that in order to obtain success in research four big 'G's were needed: Geduld, Geschick, Geld, and Gluck (patience, ability, money and luck). He was helped in his animal work by two young workers from Japan sent to train under him by Professor Kitasato in Tokyo. Kitasato had studied in Europe himself and worked with Ehrlich when he was at the Robert Koch Institute in Paris. When he returned to Tokyo he founded an Institute which he modelled on the Pasteur Institute and called 'The Tokyo Institute for Infectious Disease'. It was from here that he sent certain of his most promising young pupils to receive further training in Europe.

The first one sent to Ehrlich was Dr Shiga, who arrived in Germany in 1902 and stayed until 1905. During this time the success with Trypan red was obtained and it was through this promising result that Ehrlich was able to interest a wealthy widow, Frau Speyer, in his work. Her generosity was such that she paid for the construction of a large new building adjacent to the Serum Institute, to be used exclusively for Ehrlich's chemotherapeutic research work. In addition she provided sufficient money to pay the current expenses of the work. Thus provided with the third of his four big 'G's (Geld) he was able to extend his work considerably.

Soon after work started in the Georg Speyer Haus, Ehrlich turned his attention to an examination of arsenic and its derivatives. Workers in many parts of the world were examining the therapeutic effects of this substance at the beginning of this century. Thomas and Breinl in Liverpool discovered, in 1906, that a substance called atoxyl, an arsenical compound, had a curative action in experimental animals affected with sleeping sickness. Unfortunately it was very toxic and liable to cause blindness by its effect on the optic nerve and its use had to be abandoned. Most chemists concluded from a study of its chemical formula that it would not be possible to modify its structure, in order to produce a less toxic substance. Ehrlich decided to re-examine it, found that they were not correct and showed that it was possible to derive many other substances from it. With the help of chemists working under him, he produced altogether 606 different arsenical compounds, each of which was tested on experimentally infected animals. The one which showed great promise, once again against sleeping sickness, was No. 418—arseno-phenylglycine. Finally, Ehrlich reached his 606th preparation in 1907. His assistant who was responsible for the animal work at that time reported that it was of no use in sleeping sickness so it was therefore put on one side. Its true worth may never have been discovered had it not been that two years later, Professor Kitasato sent another young research worker to train under Ehrlich. This was Dr Hata, who for some years in Tokyo had been carrying out experiments with syphilis in rabbits. He started this work after the causative organism of the disease, which has the appearance of a spiral rod, hence its name spirochaete, had been discovered in 1905 by Schaudinn in Berlin. Hata now continued his work with Ehrlich and during the spring of 1909 systematically tried out all the compounds on rabbits infected with this disease. He was a tireless worker who patiently tested countless animals with numerous substances. He found No. 418 encouraging but continued and when at last No. 606 was reached, the results were excellent. As an adverse report about this substance had been given two years earlier, Ehrlich had it checked and rechecked before accepting his assistant's findings and allowing it to be used on human beings.

Ehrlich announced the discovery of this 606th arsenical substance at the Congress for Internal Medicine, at Wiesbaden, on 19 April 1910. He discussed the work which led to its discovery, Dr Hata described his animal experiments and Dr Schreiber of Magdeburg reported his clinical results in syphilitic patients treated with this new drug. The news was greeted by the Congress with great excitement and the Press, similarly enthusiastic, announced it to the general public in big headlines. The fact that the disease was widespread and crippling in its effect was reason enough for the public to have good cause to celebrate. What was possibly more important, was that Ehrlich had placed the search for antibacterial chemical substances on a scientific basis and had started the chain of discoveries which was to lead to the development of a succession of powerful chemo-therapeutic drugs in the twentieth century. He should not, therefore, be remembered only for his great discovery of a cure for syphilis, but also because much future success by other workers was due to the sound principles and methods initiated by him.

The world was quick to bestow appropriate honours on him. The Nobel prize had, interestingly enough, already been conferred on him in 1908, not for his work on drugs, but with Professor Metch-nikoff of the Pasteur Institute, for their work on immunity. After substance 606 was announced, universities throughout the world conferred honorary academic degrees upon him, the Prussian government made him a Privy Councillor with the title of Excellency, and the street in which his Institutes were situated, had its name changed from Sandhoff Strasse to Paul Ehrlich Strasse. All this naturally pleased him but what perhaps gave him the greatest joy was that he was elected to the very exclusive honorary membership of the German Chemical Society.

As soon as the Congress at Wiesbaden was finished visitors flocked to the Serum Institute to see Ehrlich. Patients afflicted with the disease travelled from all parts of the world asking to be cured. There were so many he could not possibly treat them himself, so he referred them to doctors who were interested in trying out the drug. These doctors were so numerous that he considered that it was fairest to give a small supply of the drug to each who asked, provided that in return he promised to report on the progress of his patients. Ehrlich also laid down strict instructions as to the method whereby the drug should be given, and stipulated that it was only to be used on cases in the early stages of the disease. As supplies at that time were strictly limited, perhaps it would have been better if he had reserved the drug for use in a few centres. By that method, carefully selected clinicians could have worked out the difficulties in the clinical use of the drug, established the best dosage and made a proper assessment of its curative power, by comparing it with a similar series of cases left untreated. This procedure is now common, for it is realized that it is the only way to assess quickly and efficiently the value of a new drug, but Ehrlich was having to deal with a problem which the medical profession had never before had to face. His method, although seemingly fair, led to a great deal of confusion and made it very difficult for him to supervise the effects of treatment. The drug could not be given by mouth but had to be injected into a muscle, which was unfortunate as most doctors at that time had little experience of the technique. Some doctors injected the substance into the superficial tissues under the skin, which caused pain, others dissolved the drug in water which had not been properly sterilized, so that infection with abscess formation developed at the site of the injection. These complications eventually led Ehrlich to insist that the drug should always be given into a vein. This was technically more difficult but he argued that it would be much safer, because any germs carelessly injected with the drug would be overcome by the defence mechanism in the blood stream. It was thought that, as this method would be more difficult for the doctors, they might not obey him, but it is of interest to note that it was generally adopted, clearly showing the high esteem in which he was held and the greatness of his authority.

The full chemical name of this 606th arsenical substance, or '606' as it was called, was dioxydiaminoarsenobenzol dihydrochloride. Obviously, it was neither possible to expect people to use this name every time they wished to refer to the drug, nor was it satisfactory for it only to be known as '606'. It therefore became known as arsphenamine, or by the trade name of Salvarsan.

A further medical congress was held the same year, this time at Königsberg, to enable all those who had been using Salvarsan to meet to discuss their results. During the five months since the congress at Wiesbaden, much work with the drug had been done and many very successful results had been obtained.

Ehrlich became involved in an incident, which on reflection is amusing, but which nearly prevented him from attending the conference. He loved Königsberg and decided, before going to the

Conference Hall, to explore the city. He misjudged the time and arrived at the congress just after the doors had been closed. He tried many side doors but without success and therefore returned to the main door and knocked loudly. The scene which ensued is well reported by his secretary, Miss Marquardt, in her biography of the great man. She says that the knocking brought along a big, dignified doorkeeper, who opened the door sufficiently to look down upon the little man outside and said, 'What do you want...Sir...?', 'Everything here is full up', and he tried to close the door again. Ehrlich however pushed and cried out loudly, 'I must get in, I must, I must get in!' The doorkeeper became angry and started to push him away, 'It is absolutely impossible, I have told you already, the hall is quite full', he shouted. The noise, by this time, had attracted the attention of some of the doctors attending the Congress, who came out to see what was happening. By now, Ehrlich had pushed the door open wide enough to get part of his body inside. 'It is this obstinate little fellow who is determined to get in', the man said. Ehrlich of course was immediately recognized by the doctors, '...but that is a very great man' one cried out, 'that is Ehrlich himself!' One can well imagine the effect this had on the poor, unfortunate doorkeeper. Ehrlich was triumphantly welcomed and enthusiastically cheered by all those present.

Following Ehrlich's pioneer discoveries, many workers adopted his methods in an attempt to discover chemical substances capable of killing disease-producing bacteria inside the body. One man who was to have outstanding success in this field was Gerard Domagk, a German, who started medical research work after the First World War. His initial efforts were not particularly successful but eventually he showed such promise that in 1927, at the age of twenty-nine, he was appointed Director of Experimental Pathology and Bacteriology, at the Elberfeld Laboratories of the large firm of I.G. Farbenindustrie. This great commercial firm was able to give all possible financial help and necessary equipment to extend his search as widely as possible.

As by this time thousands of chemical substances had been prepared in the laboratory, it might seem at first, that it must have been difficult for him to know where to start. However, he was strongly influenced by Ehrlich's success with aniline dyes and decided to explore further this group of chemical substances. Domagk was trained as a bacteriologist, so he sought the collaboration of two organic chemists, Mietzsch and Klarer, who at his request prepared a large number of azo dyes (dyes which have two linked nitrogen atoms in their molecule). He decided to study these because Eisenberg, in 1913, already had had limited success with one, a yellow dye called Chrysoidin. This killed bacteria in the laboratory, but its effect inside the body was disappointing. An even more important step had been taken in 1909, although at that time it seemed quite unrelated to the discovery of drugs, when Hörlein and others engaged in the production of new dyes for textile purposes, found that dyes were far more efficient if they contained a certain chemical combination— SO_2NH_2—the sulphonamide group. Such dyes were shown to be superior to any others because of their high degree of fastness to washing, which was produced by their extremely firm adherence to cell fibres. Mietzsch and Klarer, in the course of synthesizing hundreds of dyes therefore decided to prepare one which contained a sulphonamide group. Domagk tested this on mice infected with streptococci and found it to be extremely effective. Thus, it seemed that some property, which made the sulphonamide-containing dyes adhere firmly to textiles, caused them to behave similarly with bacteria and in so doing killed them. Therefore, he gave instructions that several substances containing this sulphonamide group should be made in order to find the one which was most effective. During the course of this search, his two chemists reviewed the various dyes already produced and decided to examine Chrysoidin which had shown such promise in 1913. In 1932 they attached a sulphonamide group to this dye to form a new chemical compound; when Domagk tested it on infected animals, the results far excelled those with any previous substance. The world knew nothing about this discovery for a further three years, until Domagk and his workers had submitted it to very carefully controlled trials. At first, it might appear that it was unfortunate that such a promising drug had to be withheld from sufferers with disease for so long, but it must be remembered that its exact therapeutic action, as well as any untoward toxic effects, had to be studied by carefully performed animal experiments before it could be used to its best advantage in man. Experience has shown that much tragedy, including death, or serious disability from unsuspected side effects, as well as shattering disillusionment from hopes unfulfilled, has been caused by drugs announced to the world too quickly. Also, it must be remembered that the drug produced by these German workers was of an entirely new type and it is to their eternal credit that, impatient as they must have been to tell the world of their success, they refrained from this until all necessary preliminary work had been completed. It was thus in 1935 that the drug was released for general medical use under the trade name of Prontosil rubrum. Immediately, from all parts of the world, reports were published of its great effect in controlling diseases such as pneumonia and particularly infection with streptococci such as occurs in puerperal fever. This disease had remained prevalent in women after childbirth even though by this time meticulous handwashing was always practised by medical students and doctors. In Great Britain alone it still killed about a thousand women every year. It had always been a particularly tragic illness because such women were usually otherwise fit and because it occurred just at a time when they had the added joy and responsibility of new-born children; therefore, there was great excitement when Colebrook and Kenny, at Queen Charlotte's Maternity Hospital in London were able to show that, by using Prontosil in women with puerperal fever, the mortality rate could be reduced from about 20 per cent to the astonishingly low figure of 4·7 per cent.

The medical profession now had a reliable drug with which to kill streptococci which cause, in addition to puerperal fever, other diseases including the one-time dreaded hospital disease, erysipelas, and the very serious disease of the tissues called cellulitis. It also had for the first time a powerful weapon to use against pneumococci which often cause one particular type of pneumonia. But there was the disadvantage that this red dye also had a poisonous effect on the cells of the body. It therefore had the somewhat paradoxical effect of making the patient feel better by overcoming the infection while at the same time making him feel ill by its toxic effects on the tissue cells. A remarkable discovery was made in France in 1936, when Trèfouel, Madame Trèfouel, Nitti and Bovet, showed that the structure of this red dye underwent change inside the body, with the production of a colourless crystalline material, called para-aminobenzenesulphonamide, and that it was this substance which was responsible for the death of bacteria. It was then realized that this chemical had already been synthesized in the laboratory, during the course of routine experiments, as long ago as 1908, but of course nobody at that time had any reason to test its action against bacteria. Ehrlich, in his quest for chemotherapeutic substances, had started with dyes only to find that his most successful discovery was not a dye but an organic arsenical substance, Salvarsan. Domagk, by following his example, started his search in the same way and discovered the highly effective red dye Prontosil, only to find that its powerful effect was not due to its properties as a dye, but because in the body it was changed into the colourless substance which is now known to the medical world as sulphanilamide. Since the discovery of this drug, scientists all over the world have been carrying out a process of molecular juggling in order to obtain others, similar in structure but more effective. This has been a long tedious business, because it has entailed replacing part of the basic structure with various organic groups, by a process of trial and error. There are many places in the sulphanilamide molecule where substitution may be made, so that countless substances have had to be tested but, by this painstaking process, many useful sulphonamide drugs have now been obtained.

The scientific world wished to show its appreciation to Domagk by awarding him the Nobel prize. This however was not to be, as is shown in an interesting paragraph in the *Manchester Guardian* of 15 December 1939 which stated 'Five Nobel prizes have just been awarded and their bestowal raises some interesting points. They are divided amongst six scientists, three of whom are German. The German Government announced at the time of the award of the Nobel Peace Prize to Herr von Ossietsky that henceforth, Germans would not be allowed to accept Nobel prizes, and according to the German Legation at Copenhagen, this ruling still applies.'

One of these Germans was Gerard Domagk. Denied this high honour by his government, he received however a much more personal reward as, in the early experimental days of Prontosil, he was able to save the life of his own daughter. She had developed a spreading cellulitis in her arm, after having pierced a finger with a needle. Every known method of treatment had been tried, without success, and it soon became obvious that the girl had not much longer to live when, as a desperate measure, some of the new and scarcely tried drug was administered. The effect was remarkable and it was not long before she made a complete recovery. It must be rare for a research scientist to benefit from his work in such a happy manner.

7

MOULDS FROM THE AIR

The next important advance was the discovery that products of certain moulds or fungi were highly effective in killing bacteria. The first one to be introduced was penicillin.

Most people now know that the discoverer of penicillin was Sir Alexander Fleming. He was born in 1881 on a farm in Scotland, the third child of a second marriage which his father entered into when he was already sixty years of age. Alexander came to London at the age of thirteen, where Tom, an elder stepbrother, had already settled as a general practitioner and they and two other brothers lived together in a house kept for them by one of their sisters. Alexander's first task in London was to continue his education at the Polytechnic in Regent Street and later found work in a shipping company in Leadenhall Street where he was paid $2\frac{1}{2}d$. an hour, while his two brothers worked in a factory producing optical lenses.

In 1900, during the Boer War, Alexander and his two optician brothers joined the London Scottish regiment. After his demobilization Alexander was unsettled and indecisive about his future. Chance, fate, or the forces of predestination according to one's philosophy, then played a strong hand in influencing events which were to lead him to become a bacteriologist at St Mary's Hospital and, thirty years later, to discover penicillin. First, by propitious timing just as he came out of the army at the age of twenty, an old bachelor uncle happened to die and left him £250 which he was persuaded by his brother Tom to use to study medicine. His future was then directed by three factors. He was undoubtedly a brilliant student, but in addition he was outstanding at swimming and shooting. He lived equidistant to three of the teaching hospitals in London, but as he had played water polo against St Mary's, and for no better reason than this, he chose that school to study medicine. After he qualified as a doctor he was given a post in the bacteriology laboratory there because, in addition to being a gifted student, he was also a crack shot! It happened that there was already on the laboratory staff a young doctor called Freeman who was most anxious to get new blood into the St Mary's Rifle Club. Fleming was planning to train as a surgeon but as there was not going to be a vacancy at St Mary's for some time it meant he would have to leave the hospital. Freeman therefore did everything he could to persuade Fleming to take up bacteriology and talked the Chief of the Department into taking him on to the laboratory staff. The chief was Sir Almroth Wright, physically a big man, with a domineering, awe-inspiring manner, who held strong beliefs and was afraid of nobody, but was one of the most dynamic and progressive medical men of that time.

One of Wright's first posts had been at the Army School of Medicine at Netley Hospital where his main interest, as for the remainder of his life, revolved around the diagnosis and treatment of infectious diseases. Widal had shown that animals could be protected against typhoid fever by the injection of dead typhoid bacilli into their blood. Wright extended this to human beings and advised the War Office to have all men going overseas inoculated against the disease. The army authorities decided they would only allow it to be done on a voluntary basis and records were so inefficiently kept that it was impossible to carry out a proper follow-up of those vaccinated so as to measure its efficacy. Wright became completely frustrated and decided that it was impossible to carry out any useful scientific work in the army medical service, so resigned. Although this must have been a depressing time for him, it was to prove beneficial both to himself and to the world in general because in 1902 he was appointed professor of pathology at St Mary's Hospital. Here he had a much greater opportunity to do original work and to carry on his lifelong ambition of finding efficient ways of combating infection. He was appalled at the helplessness of physicians at that time to influence the course of infectious diseases and stated publicly that the medical profession must find efficient means to combat infection as quickly as possible, or doctors would be forced to lose their status and become relegated to that of medical orderlies. This feeling was shared by many others and led scientists in various parts of the world to direct their energies to the problem. Metchnikoff, a Russian working at the Pasteur Institute, observed that the white cells (phagocytes) in the blood engulf and digest bacteria, and Wright felt that the key to success was to find means to stimulate the action of these phagocytes. Scientists agreed that by artificial immunization it was possible to stimulate the natural defence mechanisms in the body, including the action of the white blood cells, as a protective measure against infection. Wright argued that the same process should be used to treat infection already established. This was much contested at the time but Wright was a born fighter and was determined to prove that this was the only way to overcome infectious disease. He expressed his views forcefully and at times aggressively but, in spite of this he was revered by those under him and was deeply respected by friends in many walks of life. Amongst them were the two famous scientists Ehrlich and Metchnikoff, and the dramatist, George Bernard Shaw. The latter often listened to Wright holding forth about his theories and based his famous play, *The Doctor's Dilemma* on them.

Fleming, in contrast to his chief, was a quiet, shy, retiring Scot, who would listen attentively to his master's pontifications, but say little. His rare contributions to a discussion however, although brief, were always penetrating and apt. He had a keen analytical mind and quietly sifted the evidence without being in a hurry to express his thoughts. He agreed with Wright that immunization was an important method of treatment but felt that this was not always sufficient. He knew that infection often overcame natural defence mechanisms in the body and that to rely on the stimulation of these processes was not enough. He had seen this demonstrated forcefully and dramatically in the 1914–18 war when he had written, 'surrounded by all those infected wounds, by men who were suffering and dying without our being able to do anything to help them, I was consumed by a desire to discover, after all this struggling and waiting, something which would kill these microbes, something like Salvarsan'.

It is obvious therefore that from an early stage Fleming was looking for drugs such as had been found by Paul Ehrlich; in this, he was to obtain no help or encouragement from his chief who was almost fanatically opposed to the idea of chemical poisons. Wright had said in 1912, when addressing the Medical Research Club, that 'to use chemotherapy against bacterial infections in human beings will never be possible'. His experiences during the war did nothing to alter this view; the antiseptics available at that time, which included carbolic acid, boric acid and hydrogen peroxide, could kill bacteria outside the body but were useless against infections in wounds. They did in fact more harm than good by damaging the tissues, while at the same time giving the surgeon such a false sense of security that he became less radical and less careful in his treatment of a wound. Wright spoke forcefully about this at the time and it obviously affected his judgement for the rest of his career. He influenced those working round him and Fleming, in a Hunterian lecture in 1919, remarked that during the war opinions differed about the treatment of wounds. Some considered it more natural to rely on the body's own defences and to do everything they could to improve these, while others relied on antiseptic chemicals to poison the bacteria. He showed clearly that Sir Almroth Wright and those working with him adopted the first method. Fleming was not satisfied that the stimulation of the body's defence mechanism was sufficient and, although he appreciated that the antiseptics in current use were valueless, he was determined to continue the search for more suitable bacterial poisons.

It seems as if Fleming had an uncanny preconception that he would discover something important from the examination of old culture plates contaminated by germs in the air, which he left lying about in the laboratory. Most scientific workers would agree that it is better to keep a working bench neat and to tidy up at the end of the day so that work can be started the next day in surroundings conducive to accurate, precise and systematic work. Dr Allison, who was Fleming's colleague in the same department at St Mary's Hospital, worked like this, but Fleming teased him about his tidiness and grumbled at him for throwing culture plates away as soon as he had finished with them. Fleming always seemed to keep his culture plates lying around in an apparent jumble for weeks, although it must be admitted he always knew where to find everything. He seemed loath to part with any culture, and always before doing so examined it very carefully to see if any interesting phenomenon had occurred. It was as though he was expecting to find something important and felt that it would only be a matter of time before he did.

In 1922 he had his first triumph. He had decided to investigate the defensive properties of nasal mucus and for this purpose placed some mucus from his nose amongst a culture of bacteria. About a fortnight later he was busy one evening cleaning some culture plates which had been lying around, when suddenly he stopped because he noticed that although some large, yellow colonies of bacteria were growing as expected, there was also an area where there was no growth. He knew that this blank space was round the site where he had placed his mucus and from this observation he deduced that there must be something in the mucus which had inhibited bacterial growth. When he grew the same bacteria in broth in a test tube, the broth developed a cloudy appearance, but within a few minutes of adding some nasal mucus to the opaque suspension it cleared. Next he observed the effect of adding tears to a similar broth culture and obtained the same result. It was astonishing. After this Allison and Fleming spent much time producing tears by the painful procedure of squeezing lemon juice into their eyes and then testing the effect of the tears on various bacterial cultures. Not content with their own tears they sought donors and encouraged the laboratory workers to co-operate by paying them threepence a time! This unusual procedure was the basis of a humorous drawing in the St Mary's Hospital *Gazette* which depicted children going to the laboratory to be beaten by one attendant, while having their tears collected by another! These experiments however were extremely valuable as they showed that tears, as well as other natural secretions of the body, readily dissolved and killed certain bacteria.

As it was agreed that the substance present in these secretions must be an enzyme which dissolved (lysed) microbes, Sir Almroth Wright, who had an extensive knowledge of Greek and enjoyed constructing new words, called it lysozyme.

Fleming carried out numerous observations with lysozyme. He found that it occurred in a wide variety of tissues, not only in the respiratory tract such as in the mucus secreted by glands in the lining epithelium of the nose, mouth and trachea, but also in the blood, especially in the white cells. He also looked around at nature in general and found it in flowers such as tulips, buttercups, nettles and peonies; he found it in vegetables, an especially large amount occurring in turnips, but the richest store of all was in egg-white. Egg-white was such an easily obtainable and rich store of this substance that Fleming used it for many of his further experiments. He dis- covered that lysozyme killed most readily the various types of bacteria which are not harmful to man and that it had little effect on microbes which cause disease. He concluded from this that the only reason certain bacteria are harmless is because they are kept under control by this substance. In further experiments he showed that with a very high concentration of lysozyme, disease-producing bacteria were also killed. Elated, he felt he must be on the verge of finding a method to combat these harmful organisms. The medical world of that day however were not prepared for such a discovery, so that, when he read a paper to the Medical Research Club about the remarkable properties of this substance, it was all too obvious that nobody was interested and at the end there were no questions and no discussion. Fleming was naturally hurt but he had the quality of dogged determination to persevere in spite of the indifference of others, so with the assistance of Allison he continued the work and between 1922 and 1927 published five outstanding papers. He showed that lysozyme found in egg-white was sufficiently concen- trated to kill most bacteria in the laboratory. The next problem was to extract and purify the enzyme so that it could be used in the body. He was able to extend the work with lysozyme when Elliott Storer, who worked in his laboratory, developed in 1923 what he called a 'slide cell technique' for the purpose of studying the effect of poisons on bacteria under the microscope. The method consisted of placing two glass slides on top of each other separated by five thin strips of vaselined paper, giving four equal compartments. The compartments were filled with blood infected with bacteria, the open ends were sealed off and the apparatus placed in an incubator. The bacteria multiplied in colonies which were easy to count in the thin layer of blood between the two slides. Fleming next put various well-known antiseptics in the compartments to compare their effect both on the bacteria and on the cells in the blood. He found that every anti- septic known at that time killed the white cells far more readily than the bacteria so that it was obvious that none of them was suitable for injection into the blood stream. On the other hand, when lysozyme was placed in the compartments, it was the bacteria which were killed while the white cells were left intact. This observation led Fleming to inject an egg-white solution into a rabbit's vein which markedly increased the bactericidal power of the blood. He now believed that he possessed a useful weapon against bacteria, but realized that he would have to wait for the day when it could be purified before he could use it on human beings. This did not stop him from continuing to make valuable observations. In 1927, when he wrote his sixth paper on the subject, he described how he had found that, by adding lysozyme to a suspension of non-pathogenic bacteria in blood, most of the organisms were killed; the few that survived were removed and allowed to multiply in blood in an incubator. A higher concentration of lysozyme was then added which once again killed the majority of them. The process was repeated on several occasions with the few surviving bacteria and in this way a strain of bacteria was produced which was totally resistant to an extremely high concentration of lysozyme. Fleming had therefore now turned bacteria which were initially harmless to man into organisms which might be pathogenic. He inferred from this that lysozyme in the body had originally been an all-powerful weapon against every bacteria but that over the ages, some organisms had become resistant to it and it was these which now cause disease in man; he realized therefore that some other substance would have to be found to kill such organisms. In the meantime he tried to get a potent, purified extract of lysozyme prepared at St Mary's but he was not successful; neither Allison nor Fleming was a chemist and it is today amazing to recall that at that time St Mary's Hospital did not have a single chemist or bio-chemist on the staff to whom they could turn. In 1926 a young doctor called Ridley, who knew some chemistry, came to work in Wright's laboratory and Fleming hoped that he might be successful but they were to experience disappointment. The problem was not solved until 1937 when two chemists, Roberts and Abraham, successfully purified it in Dr Florey's laboratory at Oxford.

Fleming's experience with lysozyme however was far from wasted. Perhaps the most important aspect of the discovery was that it was a dress rehearsal in which Fleming, as the principal actor, was prepared and groomed for his role in the far more important drama which was still to be unfolded. As will be seen when his work on penicillin is discussed, the pattern of events was strikingly similar—the initial experience with the contaminated culture plate, his immediate recognition that he had made an important observation, the cool reception and indifference shown by his contemporaries, his dogged determination, his failure to find a chemist to isolate the substance, his patience and persistence against seemingly insurmountable setbacks and his final vindication when a potent antibacterial substance was purified by techniques developed in Dr Florey's laboratory at Oxford. The sequences in the two stories was so remarkably parallel that, in the midst of his work with penicillin, he must have felt at times as if he were reliving the past.

In 1928 Fleming was asked by the Medical Research Council to contribute to a book which was to be entitled *A System of Bacteriology* by writing an article on staphylococci. In preparation for this article he decided to examine a large number of culture plates on which these organisms were growing. It was necessary to take the lid off each culture plate and expose it to the air for some considerable time while he painstakingly examined it under the microscope. Then, as was his lifetime habit, he left the culture plates lying on his bench—it was as though he knew instinctively that if they became contaminated with germs from the outside air something important would happen; although he pretended it was a nuisance when they became overgrown with other germs and fungi, he always re-examined them most carefully. One day, while talking to Dr Merlin Pryce (now Professor Pryce) he took the lids off some old culture plates. He found that as usual several of them were contaminated with moulds and said ' as soon as you uncover a culture dish something tiresome is sure to happen—things fall out of the air'. He paused and after a moment added 'That's funny!' The reason for his exclamation was that, although the growth of bacteria on most of the plates was normal, some staphylococci on one plate around a particular type of mould had stopped growing so that instead of forming large, opaque, yellow masses the colonies of bacteria looked like drops of dew. Pryce, noticing Fleming's eager expression said 'That's how you discovered lysozyme'. Fleming immediately took a piece of the mould and put it into a tube of broth; at the same time he placed the dish on which the mould was growing on one side to treasure for the rest of his life.

It might be said that this event which was to lead to the discovery of penicillin had been made by chance as Fleming had not been specifically investigating the bactericidal properties of fungi but his special training had alerted his senses to the significance of the phenomenon which he observed.

He soon designed experiments to examine the properties of this mould. He grew it on an agar culture plate which he then inoculated with various types of bacteria spread out in lines radiating from the mould in the centre. He found that certain types of bacteria grew profusely at the periphery of the plate but stopped growing at the centre around the mould, whereas the growth of other types was not affected by it. He was fascinated to find that it was those types of organisms responsible for diseases in man whose growth had been most inhibited by this mould. This was a very exciting and wonderful observation and the exact opposite to the behaviour of lysozyme which he had shown killed bacteria harmless to man.

The identification of the mould at first eluded him. He consulted books on the subject and concluded that it was penicillium of the genus chrysogenum but two years later Thom, the American expert on fungi, identified it as a *Penicillium notatum*. Thom pointed out that this same fungus had originally been described by a Swedish chemist, Westling, who found it on some decayed hyssop. When Fleming heard this he was immediately reminded of the remarkable fact that David, in the seventh verse of Psalm 51 had prayed, 'Purge me with hyssop and I shall be clean'—which he considered must surely be the first known reference to its use as an antibiotic!

His next step was to culture the mould in broth, which at first was not easy. Then he filtered off the mould and carried out tests to see if the broth filtrate had any effect on bacteria. He did this by adding the liquid to various cultures of bacteria and found that it contained an active ingredient which markedly inhibited the growth of many different types of bacteria. He decided to call the bactericidal substance in the broth 'penicillin' but, because he could not yet separate it from the broth, he used the name for a time for the crude liquid. He injected $\frac{1}{2}$ c.c. into a mouse and noted that there were no side effects, and then injected 20 c.c.s into the blood stream of a rabbit, finding it no more toxic than ordinary broth. He next irrigated large surface wounds in man and the human conjunctiva on repeated occasions without any unpleasant side effects. These experiments showed that this potent, antibacterial substance, unlike any substance previously used, did little or no damage to tissue cells.

His assistant with this work was a young man named Stuart Craddock, who was to become the first patient to receive penicillin. He suffered from an infected nasal sinus from which a profuse growth of staphylococci and some haemophilus influenzae were grown. On 9 January 1929 Fleming washed out the sinus with this penicillin broth: the sinus was swabbed again three hours later and only one colony of staphylococci and a few of haemophilus influenzae were grown which showed that even this highly diluted form of penicillin had been successful in killing off most of the bacteria. However, before it could be injected into the blood stream of man it had to be separated from the broth and purified. This was to prove difficult. First Fleming turned again to the young Dr Ridley who had attempted to purify lysozyme. As the broth could not be heated for fear of inactivating the penicillin, Ridley and Craddock allowed it to evaporate in a vacuum. This left them with a brown syrupy deposit which contained concentrated penicillin; but it proved to be very unstable, and its potency quickly diminished and vanished after a fortnight. Their aim had been to produce pure crystals of this substance, but they were badly in need of expert assistance and unfortunately none was available. This was a great pity because in later years when the problem was solved at Oxford, they realized how very near to success they had been. These two young doctors then parted when Craddock married and took a better paid job at the Wellcome Research Laboratories and Ridley, ill with recurrent boils, went on a cruise. On his return he trained to be an eye specialist.

Fleming however had faith and before long persuaded Harold Raistrick, professor of biochemistry at the London School of Tropical Medicine and Hygiene, to tackle the problem. He was assisted by a young chemist called Clutterbuck and a bacteriologist named Lovell. This team came up against technical difficulties and in the midst of the work Clutterbuck died; the others carried on but were baffled by the marked instability of penicillin. All their attempts to obtain it in a potent and purified form were of no avail and they were forced to give up the struggle. Naturally, Fleming was very upset for he had fully expected this expert team to solve his problem.

Lesser men would have accepted defeat, because, in addition to his frustration about the failure to purify penicillin, Fleming felt that his fellow doctors completely lacked faith in the substance. In February 1929 he read a paper on his observations with penicillin to the Medical Research Club, but his colleagues were as coldly disinterested as when he discussed the properties of lysozyme at a similar meeting some years previously. His own chief, Sir Almroth Wright, not only failed to encourage, but actively attempted to obstruct him. In June 1929 Fleming published in *The British Journal of Experimental Pathology* a report on the present position of penicillin, and stated as part of his summing up 'it is suggested that it may be an efficient antiseptic for application to or injection into the area affected with penicillin sensitive microbes'. He had to submit this article to Wright for approval before publication and his chief was not prepared to accept this conclusion. He pointed out that he had always taught that the way to conquer infection was to stimulate the natural defence mechanisms of the body, and that Fleming himself had shown that antiseptics did more harm than good. He ordered the paragraph to be deleted but Fleming, not deterred, was prepared to fight for his belief and, although a quarrel ensued, the paragraph remained.

Gerard Domagk's discovery in 1932 of the red dye Prontosil must have been a great encouragement to Fleming. It clearly showed that an antibacterial drug could be used safely and effectively in the body, but at the same time it must have made him unhappy to think that his own substance had proved so unstable and difficult to purify. To add to his frustration he found that, when he compared the effect of the new drug from Germany with penicillin on cultures of streptococci, penicillin was very much more active. He was therefore more than ever determined to obtain a pure form of penicillin. In the meantime, Prontosil and its sulphonamide derivatives made a remarkable contribution to medicine.

As Fleming saw the wonderful results of these drugs, he might have been tempted to give up the seemingly fruitless search for ways to purify penicillin, but he knew from observations both on patients and in his laboratory, that the sulphonamides were not effective against all bacteria and that, in some cases, bacteria initially sensitive to the drug had later become resistant. His hunt for a skilled chemist therefore continued and in 1934 a biochemist named Holt attempted the task of purification but without success. Meanwhile Fleming kept his enthusiasm going by talking to his friends about his discovery. One of these was Douglas MacLeod, the gynaecologist. In 1936, during lunch, the remarkable effect of Prontosil on puerperal fever was discussed—Fleming gave much credit to the new drug but told MacLeod that he had got a substance which was much better. The fact that MacLeod, working at his own hospital, had to admit that he knew nothing about this new substance, not even its name, showed clearly what little impact Fleming's discovery had made on his colleagues. He was not upset, but with his characteristic patience and enthusiasm, discussed its potentialities just as he did at clinical meetings. The difference though was that, whereas at meetings no one bothered to ask questions, MacLeod was impressed and spent much time talking to him. Occasions like this gave Fleming much encouragement, but when about this time he asked the professor of pharmacology at St Mary's to undertake the task of extracting penicillin, he was again rebuffed; the professor showed a complete lack of enthusiasm and would not even try.

Fleming was one of the first to use Ehrlich's Salvarsan against syphilis and had followed up his patients over the years to find to his delight that they had remained cured. He predicted to Dr McElligott that penicillin would have a powerful effect on the organisms which cause both syphilis and gonorrhoea. He was later proved to be correct, but in the meantime McElligott observed the beneficial effect of sulphonamides in cases of gonorrhoea, and used to tell Fleming and Wright about this over tea. It was no surprise to Fleming for he had tested this group of drugs against gonococci in the laboratory, but Wright was maddened to think that an antibacterial agent had proved so powerful. He was certain that a vaccine would be more effective and was somewhat mollified by some experiments of Fleming with infected mice which showed that a combination of a sulphonamide and vaccine was more effective than using a sulphonamide alone. This fortunately kept the relationship between the two of them happy but there is no doubt that Wright's antagonism towards antibacterial substances delayed progress. He took no interest in sulphonamides, treated the discovery as though it had never happened and at the same time closed his mind to the possibilities of penicillin. This did not deter Fleming and in 1936, at the second International Congress of Microbiology, he demonstrated the powerful effect of penicillin on laboratory cultures of bacteria, but nobody, sad to say, showed much interest. It is possible that his dry, reserved manner and somewhat diffident mode of speech contributed to this. Although his work was not recognized in his own country, it was receiving attention in America and when he attended the third International Congress of Microbiology in New York the famous bacteriologist, Dr Dubos, asked him what had become of that promising substance called penicillin. Fleming had to confess that repeated attempts to purify it had failed and that it looked as if it wasn't worth much. At the same Congress he met another American doctor, Alvin F. Coburn, who asked many questions about lysozyme. Fleming was delighted to find that people in America had taken notice of work which had received so little attention in England.

Meanwhile at Oxford work was going on unbeknown to him. Dr Howard Florey, an Australian, was appointed to the chair of pathology at the Sir William Dunn School in Oxford in 1935. He had been interested in lysozyme for some years and soon after his appointment entrusted Dr Roberts with the task of extracting pure lysozyme, which he did in 1937. Florey decided that at the first opportunity he would have this pure substance thoroughly investigated. About this time he invited Dr E. B. Chain to Oxford to work in his biochemical department. Chain, who was born in Berlin in 1906 of a Russian father and a German mother, had qualified in Germany as a biochemist but as he was a Jew had to flee to England from the Nazis. He worked for a time with Sir Frederick Gowland Hopkins, the Director of the Institute of Biochemistry at Cambridge, who thought highly of him and recommended him to Professor Florey. Chain was delighted to obtain the post of biochemist at Oxford, for he had never expected to be given a good permanent post in England and was preparing to emigrate to Canada or Australia.

As soon as he took up his post Florey suggested to him that he might like to investigate the behaviour of the bacteriolytic substance lysozyme. This started Chain's interest in bactericidal substances in general and after completing his study of lysozyme, went through the literature to see what other work had been done on this subject. He found a large number of papers dealing with antibacterial substances and immediately became fascinated with the possibilities of microbial antagonism, or the destruction of one type of microorganism by another. He read a large number of papers on the subject but the one which interested him most was that written by Fleming in 1929 on penicillin. He read that, according to Fleming, it could destroy dangerous bacteria and was free from side effects. Chain also read that attempts had been made to purify it but that these had so far failed. He was anxious to take up the challenge but first of all money was needed. The Medical Research Council in Great Britain was sometimes prepared to give small amounts up to about £100, but knowing that this would not be nearly enough, Florey and Chain decided to ask the Rockefeller Foundation for a few thousand dollars. Chain submitted a programme of subjects to be investigated and Florey was successful in obtaining a grant of 5000 dollars for the work.

It was thus with American money that Chain started his experiments on penicillin in 1939. He had some penicillin mould at Oxford which Fleming had sent to Florey's predecessor some years ago for an entirely different research project. This had been kept and now came in useful, although Chain knew nothing about moulds and had to start from the beginning to learn how to handle them. His one advantage over Ridley and Raistrick was that the process of freeze-drying had been developed since their time and by subjecting the broth filtrate to this process he obtained a brown powder which contained penicillin with impurities. His problem now was to extract the penicillin from this. He tried to extract it with pure ethyl alcohol but failed, then to his surprise was successful with methyl alcohol and was able to obtain a small amount of partially purified penicillin. John Barnes, an assistant surgeon working with the famous Spanish surgeon, Trueta, at Oxford, injected it for him into the blood stream of a mouse without the development of any toxic effects. This was such an important finding that Florey repeated the experiment and was so surprised to find it had no effect on the mouse that he feared his injection had not gone into the blood stream. He therefore decided to repeat the experiment but to make this possible Chain had to produce more penicillin. This was no easy matter as his technique was still far from perfect, but it was well worth the effort as it confirmed that the partially purified penicillin was non-toxic. Further purification was obtained by Chain with the help of a young laboratory worker called Heatley and they set about testing its potency by placing it on culture plates adjacent to colonies of bacteria. These experiments showed that their partially purified product was one thousand times more active than crude penicillin. When eventually it was completely purified it was found to be a million times more potent than Fleming's first substance! They then devised experiments to test its effect on infections in animals. The first was on 20 May 1940 when three groups of mice were injected with three different organisms; half of them were given penicillin and half were not. Heatley sat up all night to watch with excitement as the treated mice survived while the controls all died. Next morning Florey and Chain were triumphant when they saw the result. They realized that they had in their hands an extremely valuable anti-bacterial agent which, if it could be prepared in sufficient amounts, could well make a major contribution to the recovery of sick and wounded troops. The war however was going badly, it was now June 1940, Dunkirk had fallen, and the possibility of imminent invasion of the British Isles confronted them. The Oxford team decided that they must save the miraculous mould and not allow the secret to get into the hands of the enemy: they therefore soaked the linings of their clothes in the brown liquid so that if only one escaped he would have enough mould on his person to start new cultures. In the meantime, they continued their experiments. On 1 July they injected a large number of streptococci into fifty white mice, half of them were given penicillin every three hours for forty-eight hours, the other half were left untreated as controls. Florey and his assistant were awakened by an alarm clock every two hours of the night. All twenty-five controls were dead in sixteen hours but twenty-four out of twenty-five of the mice treated with penicillin survived. It seemed almost a miracle but the result was reported soberly and factually in

The Lancet on 24 August 1940. When Fleming read the report he was both delighted and surprised as he had no idea that this work was going on in Oxford. He had asked so many chemists to purify penicillin for him, and their efforts had either failed or they had been too busy even to try. Now, when he had almost given up hope, it had been done for him without his asking. The Oxford scientists had been encouraged to do this work because of Fleming's precise accounts of the drug's potentialities in various published reports. They had not got in touch with him at any stage and, in fact, when Fleming went down to Oxford to see him, Chain had the shock of his life because he had assumed he was dead!

It was obvious to all that the time had now come to inject the drug into the blood stream of a human being. The method of purification at that time however was such that only a small amount could be made and it was essential to increase production. This was a complex problem. Florey, realizing that they would now need outside commercial help, approached the directors of a well known and very large chemical firm. These industrial chemists considered the work carefully but turned it down as their factories were already fully engaged on war work already requested by the government. Thus they were faced with the fact that when they came to test the drug on a suitable patient only a small amount was available. In February 1941 an Oxford policeman was admitted to hospital seriously ill with his blood poisoned with staphylococci, an organism which had been shown in the laboratory to be sensitive to penicillin. A small abrasion at the corner of the man's mouth had become infected and from there the staphylococci had entered the blood stream to make him a desperately ill man with abscesses all over his body. The sulphonamides had proved ineffective and he was going downhill rapidly. On 12 February 1941 he became the first patient in the world to be given pencillin in the blood stream and, within twenty-four hours, improvement was so dramatic that a dying man had been transformed into a person whose illness was under good control. Although the organisms had been reduced in number they had not been completely destroyed in so short a time and the supply of penicillin was running low. A blood transfusion was given to help build up his general resistance, also a little more penicillin, but then the supplies ran out. The bacteria immediately multiplied and the patient's condition once again deteriorated and he died on 15 March. This was a tragedy because it was obvious to all concerned that with sufficient penicillin his life would have been saved. It was a failure as an experiment too, because, since a blood transfusion had been given, critics could say that any improvement was due to this.

After further supplies had been laboriously prepared three other cases were treated. Two of these were cured and the third died from a spontaneous rupture of a blood vessel after having been brought out of a comatose state by the drug. It was clear from these results that a remarkably powerful weapon was now available against bacterial infection but, before it could be put into general use, it was necessary to produce it on a commercial scale.

Florey approached many industrial chemists but none of the big manufacturers in England at that time were in a position to take on further work. Each one was at that time fully engaged on government contracts which had to be speedily completed because the country was in a perilous stage of the war. The only alternative was once again to ask help from America, but it was not sufficient now just to ask for a loan of money, it was essential to get American industry interested in wholesale production. This led Florey and Heatley, in June 1941, to journey to the United States with some strains of the penicillium mould. This must have been an extremely anxious journey because, they were not only exposed to the hazards of a sea passage in wartime, but also they had the worry of subjecting what was well known to be a highly sensitive mould to the intense heat of an American summer. In New York, Florey met Thom who eleven years previously had first identified the mould as *Penicillium notatum*. He was now head of the section which was studying fungi at the Northern Regional Research Laboratory at Peoria, Illinois. Thom introduced him to Dr Coghill who was chief of the Division of Fermentation and the problems which confronted the English workers were put before their American colleagues. It should be mentioned that at this stage all the British secrets which had been so patiently and painstakingly amassed were fully revealed so that the work could proceed as fast as possible. At no time did any of the British workers seek to protect their discovery by taking out a patent as everyone agreed that a substance of such vital use to mankind ought not to be the subject of personal profit.

The Americans decided that the first problem was to find a suitable medium on which to grow the mould. They happened to have a large accumulation of corn steep liquor which they had been using for other work and decided to try this as a culture medium for penicillium. It proved to be a lucky choice because they quickly improved the output by more than twenty times over the amount which had been obtained at Oxford and it was soon obvious that bulk production of penicillin would be possible. At the same time it was thought that there might be other types of mould which would give a greater yield. The army authorities were asked to collect specimens from all over the world but none of these proved to have any advantage over the original mould used by Fleming. In addition however the laboratory employed a young woman whose job it was to go to the local market to buy anything mouldy that she could find, so that she soon became known as 'Mouldy Mary'! One day she returned with a mouldy cantaloup melon and it was demonstrated that this mould, which was of the *Penicillium chrysogenum* type, gave a remarkably high yield of penicillin. It is of interest that it is from moulds derived from this original one found in the decayed melon from the Peoria market place that most of our penicillin is made today.

While Heatley worked in the laboratories, Florey travelled across America and Canada trying to interest industrial chemists in the large-scale production of penicillin. As America was not yet at war the task was easier than it had been in England and he managed to find two firms willing to produce large quantities of penicillin and to send it to Oxford for research purposes.

During the time that Florey was away in the United States, Chain continued to direct the work at Oxford and his team perfected a method of extraction which enabled them to build up a small supply of the drug. The first three casualties on whom it was used were some badly burned R.A.F. pilots at the time of the Battle of Britain. A small supply was also sent to Lieut.-Col. Pulvertaft, a bacteriologist in the Military Hospital at Cairo, for use on troops of the Eighth Army. The first man to have the benefit of it there was a young New Zealand officer suffering from widespread infection complicating a compound fracture of his leg. He had a high fever and was desperately ill with his sheets soaked with the pus which dripped from his wounds. When he had been ill for six months and was dying, small rubber tubes were put into the infected tissue in the left leg and a very weak solution of penicillin instilled. Within ten days the leg had healed and after a month he was back on his feet. Pulvertaft had enough penicillin for ten similar cases, nine of which made complete recoveries.

These were exciting and momentous days for doctors who had become used to watching men with badly infected wounds gradually succumb, in spite of all their efforts. Everyone was full of praise for this new substance and for the workers at Oxford who had produced it. It seemed for a time as if Alexander Fleming, whose sagacity and perseverance had made all this possible was to be overlooked and forgotten. His old chief, Sir Almroth Wright, however took the opportunity to compensate for his lack of enthusiasm in the early days, when he reminded the world of the man who made the discovery and to whom it owed an enormous debt of gratitude. This opportunity occurred after Fleming had saved the life of a friend who had been admitted to St Mary's Hospital seriously ill with an infection of the meninges—the membranes which cover the brain and spinal cord. This meningitis was due to an infection with a streptococcus which Fleming had demonstrated in the laboratory was not affected by sulphonamides, but was sensitive to penicillin. He therefore telephoned Florey to explain the situation, although the patient was comatose and the position seemed almost hopeless. Florey sent him a little of his precious reserve of the drug and on the evening of 6 August 1942, the first injection was given into the blood stream. Some improvement occurred but examination of the cerebrospinal fluid which circulates between the meninges showed that the penicillin was not getting to the infected part in a sufficiently high concentration. It was then decided to inject the penicillin for the first time through a needle directly into the man's cerebrospinal fluid. This was done with some trepidation as Florey had tried it out on a cat which had promptly died, but a similar injection into the man had no ill effects and he made a miraculous recovery.

This success caused great excitement, was widely discussed in medical circles and on 24 August 1942 *The Times* published a leading article entitled 'Penicillium'. It spoke of its virtue and pointed out that the substance was a hundred times more potent than sulphonamides but was difficult to make. It urged that in view of its importance every effort should be made to find methods of providing large quantities of the drug as soon as possible. It almost amounted to an order to the British government that, as part of the war effort, it should see that sufficient of it was made, but no reference was made to the pioneer work which was being done by the Oxford team, or to Fleming. Sir Almroth Wright may have lacked initial enthusiasm and been slow to give encouragement during the time that Fleming was studying the penicillium mould but, now that victory had been attained, he was not going to stand by and allow the world to reap the benefits of penicillin, without due recognition being given to the man who discovered it. He therefore wrote a letter to *The Times* published on 31 August, in which he pointed out that in the paper's recent leading article on penicillin it had refrained from putting a laurel wreath for the discovery round anybody's brow and made it clear that it was to Fleming that this honour was due. In view of the fact that he had been so hostile towards any suggestion that infection could be controlled by chemotherapy, it must have taken much moral courage to come forward, at the age of eighty-one, to support his junior colleague.

Fleming and Florey corresponded frequently and planned to mass produce penicillin in Britain. Fleming therefore went to see Sir Alexander Duncan, the Minister of Supply, who decided that a committee should be set up in Britain under the direction of Sir Cecil Weir, the Director-General of Equipment. On 28 September 1942 he summoned a conference at Portland House in London to include Fleming, Florey, Raistrick and representatives of chemical and pharmaceutical industries. Everyone attended in a most co-operative spirit and it was unanimously agreed by all concerned that the work must be done without any ulterior motive of personal gain and that all secrets must be shared so that the drug could be made available as quickly as possible for the treatment of the sick and wounded.

In the United States, progress was slow at the start, but all the workers were most enthusiastic and, before long, the technical difficulties had been overcome and large quantities were released. By 1943 sufficient stocks were available to supply the armed forces and by the following year there was plenty available for civilians as well.

The world now hastened to pay homage to the little Scot whose work in the laboratory at St Mary's Hospital had led to such a miraculous discovery. In 1943 he was elected a Fellow of the Royal Society, the highest honour his brother scientists could bestow upon him. In July 1944 he received the accolade from King George VI of Knight Bachelor.

As Professor Sir Alexander Fleming he lived another eleven years during which time he was able to watch the revolution in medicine brought about by his discovery.

8

MOULDS FROM THE SOIL

While young Fleming was playing in the fields around his father's farm in Scotland, another boy, who was to make a similar and equally important contribution to medical science, was growing up in a humble home in the isolation of the Russian Ukraine. His name was Selman Waksman. His birth on 8 July 1888 could hardly have been less propitious. His birthplace was the bleak, small town of Novaia-Priluka where the inhabitants lived in primitive, white-washed, straw-thatched houses. They were for the most part poor because, although the soil was very fertile and the crops plentiful, all the profits went to the landlords, the Czar and the police. It was a land filled with dissatisfaction, distrust and corruption. The peasants in Russia at that time had been liberated from slavery about forty years previously, but they still had much cause for bitterness, and the revolution was in the making. Waksman's family was Jewish and the Jews existed in a state of uneasy truce with the rest of the population.

Waksman's father had inherited some land but was not particularly industrious and although Selman liked him, they had no interests in common. His mother, on the other hand, was a bright, dynamic person who was his inspiration, and during his childhood they were devoted to each other. Their attachment was made closer by the fact that he was an only child, except for a brief period at the age of seven when he had a sister, who lived for less than two years.

He attended the local school and in addition his mother arranged for him to have some private tuition at home. He was quick to learn and by the age of thirteen, encouraged by his mother, he began to teach others and organized a school to teach children who otherwise would have remained without any education. For a time he lived a happy life at home with his mother, but this was not to last, because as he reached maturity the country was plunged into the disastrous Russo-Japanese war of 1904 to 1905. This had far-reaching consequences and awakened the people to a realization of their miserable existence, and revealed to them how corrupt and rotten was their government and the extent to which they were exploited by the rulers. Organized protests and general strikes developed and the Czar was forced to promise improvements. No sooner had he done this than the police and cossacks raided the towns and arrested leaders of the revolution, shooting some and deporting others to Siberia. The suppression was ruthless and many innocent people lost their lives.

The little town of Priluka was not directly involved, but Waksman realized that the spirit of disunity which had split the country was bound to affect him sooner or later. He was therefore determined to complete his education as quickly as possible before everything became too disorganized. He left home to continue his studies in the bigger cities. Examinations were difficult because of the strong bias against Jews but his work was of such outstanding merit that the authorities were forced to pass him.

This antagonism to the Jews was expressed not only in everyday life, but also in the official attitude of school authorities. Many schools would only take a son of Jewish parents on condition that they not only paid for their child, but also for a non-Jewish boy as well. Jewish teachers too did not escape from this tyranny and one of Waksman's most successful teachers, a hunchback who taught mathematics, physics and chemistry, had to organize his own evening school because no university or school would employ him. This meant that he was deprived of laboratory facilities and could not give practical demonstrations in chemistry and physics, but he was devoted to his work and managed to hold the attention of his class with the help of a blackboard alone.

Waksman was nearing the end of his school studies when, without warning, he suffered a most grievous blow which was radically to affect his future. In the summer of 1909 while he was at home on holiday, his mother suddenly developed an obstruction of the bowel for which an immediate operation was necessary. This was only possible in a large hospital and they had to undertake an overnight train journey to Kiev. By the time she reached hospital, his mother's condition was too poor for her to stand up to an operation. Her son never left her, while for two weeks her condition gradually deteriorated.

At her death he felt himself completely alone, for although his father and cousins were there, they were of little account.

He decided that he must move as quickly as possible from the neighbourhood where he had so many memories of his mother and, in the autumn of 1909, he and a friend returned to Odessa to continue their studies. In the following year he passed his final examination which permitted him to enter university. He was anxious not to go to a university in Russia, as entrance to these institutions for Jews was strictly limited, the country was becoming increasingly unhappy and divided, with the people living in fear of the Czar and his brutal police, while the future for Jews was particularly black. Above all, the one person to whom he was deeply attached had died, so he decided to emigrate and start a new life elsewhere. Some of his cousins had already settled in America and wrote persuading him to join them. He left Europe in the middle of October 1910 on his journey to the New World. He was over twelve days in the steerage accommodation of a small ship, where he shared a meagre diet of herrings and boiled potatoes, or boiled beef and black bread with several hundred other youthful emigrants. His boat arrived on 2 November 1910 in Philadelphia, where he was met by two of his cousins. One of them, Mendel Kornblatt, took him to his farm at Metuchen in New Jersey, where he stayed for some time. This cousin was to have a great influence on Selman's future. He showed him the problems of farm life, and gave him instructions in the basic principles of plant and animal growth, and the influence exerted on this by environment, nutrition and heredity. He taught him how best to prepare and use compost, the proper selection of seeds, the art of growing vegetables and the technique of rearing chickens. Waksman had a scientific type of mind and was delighted to find that his cousin was able to introduce him to all the fundamental chemical and biological aspects of agriculture. It encouraged him to want to learn more about the chemical reactions which occur in living bodies so he decided he ought to become a student at a university. At first he thought that he could best be trained in the subject at a medical school but at the suggestion of his cousin he visited Rutgers College, New Brunswick, only a few miles away from the farm. There he discussed his future with another immigrant from Russia, Dr Jacob Lipman, head of the

Department of Bacteriology, and soon to become Dean of the College of Agriculture. Lipman persuaded him to apply for training at his college.

With the help of a scholarship gained in a State competitive examination he began work as an agricultural student at Rutgers in September 1911. It was not easy for him to work and compete with other students in this new country, with its language which was strange to him and its very different social pattern. He found the American students were not very helpful and at times laughed at his difficulties with their language, but he was determined to let nothing deter him. He was fortunate in having some inspiring teachers to instruct him in chemistry, physics, biology, bacteriology and all the various branches of scientific agriculture. For the first two and a half years at the university he continued to live on his cousin's farm. This had the advantage that he was able to earn his keep by helping with the work there but it did also mean that he was not able to read his books as much as he would have liked. He therefore moved to New Brunswick so that he could be nearer to the university, and to keep himself alive took on various spare-time jobs including teaching English to foreign immigrants. As his course in agriculture proceeded he developed a particular interest in the study of the soil and, as he had made extremely rapid progress during his course, he was excused from attending formal classes during his last year and was able to devote himself to a research project. The subject he chose was an enumeration of the different types of micro-organisms to be found in the soil. It was this study, initiated during his last year of student life, which was to lead him years later to the discovery of streptomycin. Nobody could have anticipated that such an important contribution to medicine would come from a study of the soil, and certainly Waksman's early interest was entirely academic.

In this study he dug trenches in the college farm each month of the year and observed that there were various quite distinct soil layers at different depths. He took samples of soil from each layer under aseptic conditions and cultured them on special culture media. He found that the most plentiful organisms were colonies of bacteria but that colonies of moulds or fungi were also scattered about. In addition, to his great surprise, he noted an abundance of small colonies which to the naked eye looked like bacteria but under the microscope had the appearance of fungi. When he drew the attention of his teachers to these he found they did not know much about them. After further study Waksman came to the conclusion that they were representatives of what was then an obscure group of microbes called actinomycetes, or Ray fungi, so-called because of the characteristic radiating pattern of their structure under the microscope. It had been known for some thirty years that varieties of this group could cause the disease actinomycosis in man and in cattle; it is interesting to note that this is successfully controlled today by penicillin, which is itself derived from a fungus. This is therefore a good example of the way man has learned to counteract the ill-effects of one fungus by the action of another.

It was from a variety of these actinomycetes that Waksman at a later date produced streptomycin. He little knew when his interest was first focused on them what an important part they were to play in his life, but for some compelling reason he found that he was to make a close study of them over many years, and that it was to remain his major scientific interest for the rest of his life.

He graduated with a Bachelor of Science degree in 1915. His teacher of botany, Dr Halsted, appreciated his abilities and offered him a post in his department. Waksman felt that his primary interest was not in general botany but in a specialist study of the soil and its life, especially in the little understood actinomycetes. This fundamental desire to study the mysteries of the soil must have been subconsciously developing in his mind since the days of his childhood spent amongst the highly productive fertile black earth of the Russian Ukraine and that every step he had taken since had been directed towards this. So he turned down Halsted's offer and discussed his ambitions with Dr Lipman who had taught him soil bacteriology. As soon as Dr Lipman knew of his particular interest he was appointed as research assistant in soil bacteriology at the New Jersey Agricultural Experimental Station, an Institution with which he was to be associated for most of his future life.

On taking up his new job he lost no time in beginning his study of the actinomycetes and was soon ready to publish an account of his observations, which he did in February 1916. From this work he attained the higher degree of Master of Science but also gained much more than academic distinction, for it led him to formulate certain basic principles, which were to guide him throughout his scientific career to the final triumph of his great discovery. As an undergraduate he had already shown, from his soil sampling of trenches, that bacteria, fungi and actinomycetes differed in their distribution throughout the various depths of soil. The number of bacteria diminished steadily from the surface of the soil downwards, whereas the number of actinomycetes diminished more slowly with increasing depth so that their proportion gradually increased from about 10 per cent on the surface to something like 70 per cent at a depth of 30 inches. He came to the conclusion that micro-organisms live in a somewhat complex community. Some are helpful by providing their neighbours with food but others are destructive, either by consuming those around them, or by otherwise interfering with their growth.

While continuing to observe the distribution of actinomycetes in the soil, he made a careful study of their biochemical and physiological activities. During this time, he realized that he rarely came across any disease-producing germs in the soil. This he considered to be very strange, for he was well aware that a large number of organisms infect man, animals and plants, and that these must at some time find their way into the soil, either in excreta or from dead animals. He observed that such organisms tended to disappear rapidly in the soil and asked himself whether it was because they were unable to live in this environment or because they were destroyed by other soil microbes. If the latter were true he wondered if soil microbes could be used to combat disease in man. Other people were having similar thoughts and in 1927 Dr Avery of the Rockefeller Institute asked him to recommend a good man trained in soil microbiology, who could attempt the isolation of an organism from the soil capable of destroying the pneumococcus. Waksman suggested that René Dubos, a young Frenchman who was working in his laboratory at that time, might like to try. By 1932 Dubos managed to isolate a soil bacillus which had the power to destroy the envelope or capsule around the pneumococcus, making it vulnerable to attack by the white cells in the blood stream.

The same year that Dubos made this discovery, Waksman was

asked by the National Research Council and the Tuberculosis Association to study the fate of tubercle bacilli in the soil. One of his assistants confirmed, what had in fact been previously shown, that tubercle bacilli do not remain alive for very long there. It was thought possibly that this was because they were attacked by organisms already present in the soil. Waksman therefore encouraged Dubos to study this problem. In 1939, as the result of this investigation, Dubos isolated a substance called tyrothricin from soil bacteria, which had the power to destroy pathogenic organisms. It did not prove to be an ideal therapeutic substance but his discovery was of great importance, as it clearly demonstrated to Waksman that this line of research was worth while.

Before long Waksman and his team turned once again to the actinomycetes and in 1940, from a culture of one variety, he isolated an active substance which he called actinomycin. This proved to be highly toxic to animals, and they therefore continued to examine systematically other varieties of actinomyces as well as countless other types of micro-organisms. The work was extremely tedious as it involved not only finding which organisms produced chemical substances, but also the conditions of growth which gave the best yield. It was then necessary to test the inhibitory power of the chemical extracts against various types of organisms, both pathogenic and non-pathogenic. The promising ones had to be further purified and concentrated, before their toxicity to animals could be assessed. This was followed by a study of their effect on germs in animals and, finally, the most promising of them had to be tested against pathogenic organisms in man. This outline of the steps that had to be taken indicates something of the enormity of the task on which the team was engaged. Waksman and his assistants had to face numerous disappointments but by 1942 they had isolated another substance called streptothricin which, although less toxic than actinomycin, had very definite limitations. The search therefore continued and in 1943 their efforts were rewarded when streptomycin was extracted from *Actinomyces griseus*. Although streptomycin was shown to have toxic effects it was soon obvious that it was extremely effective against a large number of organisms pathogenic to man.

It is of interest to note that this particular organism, *Actinomyces griseus*, had been isolated by Waksman and Curtis in 1915 but that, at that time, their minds were not alive to the possibilities of any antibacterial effect which it might have had, and so of course no suitable tests were devised. By the time streptomycin was isolated a total of about one hundred thousand different cultures of various types had been examined. It had therefore been a gigantic task. Of all the different organisms, the actinomycetes had produced the highest number of promising substances, and since then have been the source of other valuable antibiotics.

After the isolation of streptomycin, it was soon apparent that a discovery had been made of similar importance to that of penicillin and, further, that this drug was a powerful weapon against many microbes not affected by penicillin.

Tuberculosis had for centuries been a major cause of death in man and everyone hoped, as each new drug was discovered, that a cure had at last been found. Waksman therefore lost no time, early in 1944, in exposing tubercle bacilli on culture plates to streptomycin and soon found that their growth was markedly inhibited. Shortly after, Dr Feldman and Dr Hinshaw at the Mayo Clinic in Rochester, Minnesota, demonstrated that it was effective in guinea-pigs infected with tuberculosis and that the drug had a favourable effect on tuberculosis in man. Several industrial companies became interested in its manufacture and by 1946 a rapid reduction in price made possible the wide use of the drug. It is now well known that many people who would otherwise have died from tuberculosis owe their lives to the discovery.

9

THE WHITE PLAGUE

Tuberculosis has been one of man's main enemies for centuries and, although a certain amount of control was achieved by improved hygiene, sanitation and housing in some parts of the world during the earlier part of this century, there was no hope of successfully conquering it until the introduction of effective chemotherapy after the Second World War. Previously treatment usually gave only temporary benefit so that the disease often recurred and ultimately proved fatal. Due to the use of potent drugs during the past ten years, the mortality rate has been falling rapidly in most highly developed countries although the disease is still widespread in those parts of the world where the drugs are scarce or badly used.

The discovery of streptomycin and its powerful effect against the tubercle bacillus was a great therapeutic advance, but it was soon realized that it was of very limited value when used by itself. When first given to a patient the effect on the disease was remarkable: the patient's general condition rapidly improved, and X-rays of the lungs showed surprisingly rapid clearing of abnormal shadows. But after some weeks, it was found that it began to lose its effect and finally became useless. The reason for this is that tubercle bacilli in some way adapt themselves to streptomycin and become resistant to its action, so that they are no longer killed, but continue to multiply in its presence. This development by bacteria of what is called 'drug resistance' is not confined to the action of streptomycin on tubercle bacilli, but also occurs with many other antibiotics in their action on other organisms. This big problem is seriously affecting man's conquest of many bacterial diseases, but in the case of tuberculosis a way to overcome the difficulty with streptomycin has fortunately been discovered.

While Waksman was at work on soil fungi, other scientists were experimenting with various chemical substances, and testing them, by a method of trial and error, against the tubercle bacillus. Usually there was no clue as to which might prove effective, so that the work was laborious and time-consuming. In 1941 Bernheim gave a definite lead when he noted that salicylates suppressed the growth of tubercle bacilli on laboratory culture plates, by interfering with their oxygenation. Lehmann in Sweden followed up Bernheim's clue by testing a large number of different salicylic acid compounds against tubercle bacilli in the laboratory and found that para-aminosalicylic acid (P.A.S.) was the most promising. Next he administered it to guinea-pigs and rats to check for any toxic reactions and finally considered it was safe to give it to patients.

In March 1944 twenty tuberculous patients in Gothenburg were given the drug. It was reported that their general condition improved, with reduction of fever, increased appetite and gain in weight. It was soon found however that by itself its effect on tuberculosis in man was not as good as had been initially supposed, and at one stage it looked as if its use might be abandoned. Fortunately, as it was discovered about the same time as streptomycin, it was not long before the two drugs were used in combination. To everyone's surprise, it was found that when the two were given together, streptomycin no longer lost its effect after a short time because of the development of bacterial resistance, but could be profitably administered for many months. This was probably the most important step in the battle against tuberculosis. Much work had still to be done to determine the optimum dosage for these two drugs and the length of time for which they should be given. It was found that if the daily dose was too big there were serious toxic side effects, but that it was necessary to continue treatment for many months in order to avoid relapse.

Until then, when any new drug had been discovered, separate small trials had been carried out by individual physicians on a limited number of patients, which meant that no one could gain more than a clinical impression as to the efficacy of the substance. Initial pilot studies to assess the value of streptomycin against tuberculosis were done at the Mayo Clinic in America, and the results published in 1944. Following this, however, and for the first time in medical history, large scientifically controlled trials were organized in Great Britain by the Medical Research Council in co-operation with the

Research Committee of the British Tuberculosis Association, and in America by the Veterans Administration, the United States Public Health Service and, in the early phase, by the American Trudeau Society. Hundreds of patients with widespread, rapidly progressive tuberculosis of the lungs were admitted into these trials. Half were given the standard orthodox treatment of that time, and the other half were given the new drugs. The progress of the two groups was then compared, both by clinical examination and radiological assessment, and in this way it was possible to measure exactly and quickly the advantages and any disadvantages, of these new drugs. At the same time, by dividing the main groups into sub-groups, a comparison could be made as to the efficacy of various treatment regimes, the optimum dosage and duration of treatment.

The result of the first trial in this country using streptomycin by itself was published jointly by the Medical Research Council and the British Tuberculosis Association in 1948. Following this, similar controlled trials were carried out using para-aminosalicylic acid (P.A.S.) alone and also using the two drugs simultaneously. The final results were published in November 1950, but at the end of 1949 the enormous advantages of using the two drugs together in the prevention of streptomycin resistance became obvious. It was not felt justifiable therefore to withhold this information until the trial had been formally completed, so an interim communication was published in the British medical press in December 1949, and a similar report, by American workers, was published in the American Review of Tuberculosis in the same year. This was the most important observation ever made in the treatment of tuberculosis, and a turning point in the history of man's fight against the disease. It still meant that patients needed many months of treatment, but it enabled streptomycin to assert its powerful effect over long periods, and thus gradually but surely to kill the millions of tubercle bacilli living and dividing in diseased tissue.

At the same time as these drugs were being used in hospital wards, work was going on in the laboratory to find other drugs which might prove to be even better. After Domagk discovered Prontosil, a large number of sulphonamide drugs were produced and tested systematically against the tubercle bacillus. None proved to be particularly powerful, but one or two showed sufficient promise to lead Domagk to examine other chemical substances with similar structures. In this way, twelve years after his original discovery of Prontosil, he was able to show that an entirely new group of substances, the thiosemicarbazones, had a marked inhibitory effect on the tubercle bacillus in the laboratory. Although they were not to prove of great value in the treatment of tuberculosis, they nevertheless were of great importance, because it was from a systematic study of them that scientists were eventually led to examine the effect of various derivatives of nicotinic acid. One of these, isonicotinic acid hydrazide (isoniazid) was to prove outstandingly useful.

Isonicotinic acid hydrazide had been synthesized in the laboratory by Hans Meyer and Josef Mally as long ago as 1912, at a time when people were willing to believe in anti-microbial therapy following the introduction of arsphenamine by Ehrlich less than two years previously, but unfortunately no one was then looking for an anti-tuberculous drug. On the other hand, by the middle of this century, in the light of success already attained, many research centres were actively looking for anti-tuberculous compounds. By 1951 three independent pharmaceutical firms, Hoffmann la Roche, Squibb and Bayer, knowing nothing of each other's work, had undertaken a study of isomers of nicotinic acid, as a direct result of systematic work on the thiosemicarbazone group. Each firm separately concluded that isoniazid showed such promise that it must be tried out on human beings, so they approached three different clinical centres; Hoffmann la Roche went to Drs Robitsek and Selikoff at the Seaview Hospital, Staten Island, New York; Squibb approached Professor Walsh McDermott at Cornell University; and Bayer went to Professor Klee at Elberfeld. A situation therefore arose whereby three medical centres were conducting clinical trials on the same drug, each one unaware that there were others doing similar work. Professor McDermott has described an amusing incident which occurred when Gerard Domagk visited his laboratory on 28 September 1951. Considerable discussion took place on the subject of anti-tuberculous drugs in general, and the thiosemicarbazones in particular. Neither however mentioned that he was taking part in a clinical trial of isoniazid, and in retrospect McDermott feels certain that each one must have walked away from their meeting with the thought, 'Isn't he in for a surprise'. In fact they were both to have a big surprise because neither knew of the existence of the Hoffmann la Roche clinical trial which Drs Robitsek and Selikoff had already started. Nevertheless, the three groups came eventually together, and arrangements were made for publication of the results in scientific journals in the first week of April 1952. Unfortunately a highly dramatized and sensational account exploded in the lay press some time before this, telling the world that at last a miracle cure had been discovered for tuberculosis. As a result sufferers all over the world began to demand this drug before it had been properly assessed. A leading article in *The Lancet* on 5 April 1952, drawing attention to this, stated that it was most unfortunate that such sensational statements had been made, because, as the drug could be produced cheaply in large quantities and was easy to take, it would be a great temptation for physicians to prescribe it for all tuberculous patients, whether in hospital, or at home without adequate supervision or safeguards. It pointed out that in America general distribution had not yet been authorized, and it hoped that the profession in this country would be no less careful. It stated that there were very real risks in the widespread and uncontrolled use of drugs before they have been properly evaluated, particularly in the case of this drug, as it was not yet known whether drug resistance would develop, as had happened with streptomycin. In the summer the Ministry of Health also issued a similar statement. In spite of these warnings, the drug was given by itself to thousands of tuberculous patients, and in every case the tubercle bacilli became resistant to the drug so that it ceased to be effective after a few weeks. The results of clinical trials showed that it retained its power for very long periods, providing it was prescribed with either streptomycin or para-aminosalicylic acid.

It has therefore become an established practice always to prescribe these drugs in combination, either in pairs or sometimes all three together. Further, it has been found essential to continue daily treatment for about two years in the majority of cases. Unfortunately, it has been found difficult to persuade certain people to take the drugs regularly, and in the prescribed combination. The result is similar to taking one drug by itself, with the development of tubercle bacilli resistant to the drugs, so that not only does their disease become untreatable, but also other people are liable to be infected with these dangerous organisms. This problem is particularly common in many underdeveloped countries, and is seriously impeding the eradication of the disease. The search for other effective drugs continues, and already a few have been discovered, but they all have the disadvantage of unpleasant toxic side effects which seriously limits their use.

10

VICTORY AND ITS AFTERMATH

During recent years there has been the greatest change in the pattern of disease that the world has ever seen. Today it is taken for granted that most disease-producing microbes can be killed by one drug or another. This is remarkable when it is considered that at the beginning of the century, with the exception of one or two diseases, there was no effective treatment, and even in the years leading up to the Second World War it was commonplace for parents to have to face losing a child through some bacterial disease and for young adults to succumb to infection just as they were starting their careers. Medical wards in hospitals always had a large number of young people seriously ill with diseases such as pneumonia, meningitis and septicaemia, while the air in the surgical wards was filled with the stench of uncontrolled pus which discharged from carbuncles, abscesses and festering wounds. Now all this is changed, due to the discovery of sulphonamides, penicillin, streptomycin and, more recently, a further large range of drugs including tetracycline, chloramphenicol, erythromycin and novabiocin. This last group of drugs was discovered by a prolongation of the search amongst the actinomycetes initiated by Waksman.

Man however has not had, and is not likely to have in the future, everything his own way. Some bacteria have learned to resist the action of these substances and to become drug resistant. Fortunately, up to now, when resistance develops to one drug another effective one is usually available. A good example of this may be seen in our experience with staphylococci. This germ was initially nearly always killed by penicillin but in recent years strains of it have become resistant to this drug. Chloramphenicol, erythromycin and novabiocin were introduced in time to deal with these resistant staphylococci and now, when strains are appearing which are resistant to these drugs other effective analogues of penicillin have been discovered. Another example may be found in the treatment of gonorrhoea—some years ago all gonococcal infections were quickly controlled with penicillin but in recent years some gonococci have become resistant to it, and other drugs have had to be used. It can therefore be seen that, in the continuous conflict between man and bacteria, man has so far managed to keep one move ahead but it will be essential to continue to find new drugs if he is to retain the mastery.

Fortunately some bacteria do not develop drug resistance, for instance the pneumococcus—a common cause of pneumonia—remains easily killed by penicillin, as is the streptococcus frequently found in throat infections and the spirochaete responsible for syphilis.

As the mortality from bacterial disease today is low, death for countless people is deferred, but once old age is reached this ready control of infection may be a disadvantage; pneumonia at one time was the 'old man's friend' as it brought life to an end in a state of toxic confusion, but too often now people are robbed of this merciful release and continue to survive although the strength to enjoy an active life has gone. At the moment there is a large number of pathetic elderly people who exist in a state of loneliness and neglect, and this situation will become more acute when a cure for cancer is discovered. Already some promising drugs have been found for various forms of malignant disease and it is certain that with all the thought that is being put into this problem, one day in the near future a chemical to kill cancer cells will be discovered. This will lead to a further increase in the proportion of old people.

The increased life span which has already resulted from the control of bacterial infection has led to a great expansion in the population of the world. In highly developed communities this effect has been partly counteracted by the use of contraceptives to control family size. Large families today result in marked overcrowding and add to the already great problem of insufficient housing. Restriction of family size in the changed circumstances of life expectation is obviously intelligent though there are theoretical objections to the artificial control of population, as this reduces the chances of potential fine stock, at a time when some of the weakest are kept alive by the advances in modern medicine. It also means that the relative proportion of young people in the community will decrease while the number of elderly will increase. In practice, however, these disadvantages are not of primary importance in an affluent society because, with modern advances in the fields of technology, it needs relatively few to work to be able to feed and look after the others. Amongst poorer communities, where the supply of food is limited, population control is of paramount importance in order to prevent famine and starvation. This means that people in countries with a very high birth-rate such as in the Far East must be suitably educated, and if necessary given financial assistance, so that everything possible is done to encourage them to adopt efficient contraceptive techniques. It is unfortunate that present mechanical methods are clumsy and, without proper care, inefficient, and thus are ill-suited for use by under privileged people. It is therefore with a sense of urgency that the efficiency of chemical hormones taken by mouth is being tested. These are simple to take, and so far appear to be effective, but it is too early to say whether or not they will have any unfortunate side effects after prolonged use.

It has to be faced that although man's conquest of bacterial disease has brought much individual happiness, it has had far-reaching social implications, and it may prove to be a mixed blessing unless every community takes positive steps now to reduce their birth-rate in the light of these changed circumstances. In 1900 the world population was about 1600 million: today it has nearly doubled that figure and at the end of this century, with the present rate of increase, it is expected to have trebled or quadrupled so as to be between 5000 million and 7000 million. There is evidence that governments throughout the world have already become acutely aware of this problem; India has spent three million pounds on a birth-control campaign but up to now its effects have been negligible. In Japan there has been greater success and its birth-rate has dropped considerably in recent years. This however is mainly due to voluntary sterilization and abortion, rather than to the use of contraceptives. In 1956 there were 1,160,000 sanctioned abortions. It is strange for those in the western world who have been brought up to consider abortion and sterilization, except for strictly limited medical indications, as criminal, to have to face now that in certain parts of the world these operations have not only to be condoned, but actively encouraged. It was unfortunate, and looked as if it might have much significance for the western world, when the Communist government in China withdrew its support for family planning at the beginning of the country's 'great leap forward' programme of economic expansion in 1958. The official attitude was that it was only capitalist countries which need fear over-population, although this was not the opinion of Russian politicians, including Khrushchev. Since then the leaders in China must have changed their minds because in 1962 birth control once again became officially sponsored, and the Chinese government has now launched a vigorous campaign against early marriage. Young couples have been told that the wife should wait until she is in her middle twenties before having her first child, and that further children should be spaced at intervals of three to five years. In order to assist with this Chinese newspapers have recently published detailed descriptions of various types of contraceptives available. The wisdom of this policy becomes apparent when it is appreciated that the present population of China is believed to be about 680 million and is increasing at the rate of at least 12 million every year.

If it is accepted that the world will have to control strictly the number of births in the future, a case could be made also for the control of their quality, by adoption of methods of artificial selection, such as is already being done with animals and plants. Fortunately this is abhorrent to most people, who feel that to interfere with nature to this extent, would not only be unnecessary but wrong, for it would too radically interfere with man's liberty and individuality.

At the close of a book dealing with so many of man's triumphs over disease, it is unfortunate to have to show that these have produced their own problems which, unless wisely handled, can lead to as much misery as did the diseases themselves. As was aptly said in *The British Medical Journal* recently, 'even if the human species retains sufficient control over its aggressive instincts to prevent a catastrophic war, can its reproductive instincts be curbed to avoid terrible hardship?'

INDEX